Changing Values in Medical and Health Care Decision Making

Changing Values in Medical and Health Care Decision Making

Edited by

Uffe Juul Jensen
Aarhus University
Denmark

and

Gavin Mooney
University of Copenhagen
Denmark

JOHN WILEY & SONS
Chichester · New York · Brisbane · Toronto · Singapore

Distributed in the United States of America, Canada and Japan by Alan R. Liss Inc., 41 East 11th Street, New York, NY 10003, USA.

Other Wiley Editorial Offices

John Wiley & Sons, Inc., 605 Third Avenue,
New York, NY 10158-0012, USA

Jacaranda Wiley Ltd, G.P.O. Box 859, Brisbane,
Queensland 4001, Australia

John Wiley & Sons (Canada) Ltd, 22 Worcester Road,
Rexdale, Ontario M9W 1L1, Canada

John Wiley & Sons (SEA) Pte Ltd, 37 Jalan Pemimpin 05-04,
Block B, Union Industrial Building, Singapore 2057

Library of Congress Cataloging-in-Publication Data

Changing values in medical and health care decision making / edited by Uffe Juul Jensen and Gavin Mooney.
p. cm.
Book originated in an international conference held at the University of Aarhus, Denmark, in June 1988.
The conference was sponsored by the European Society for Philosophy of Medicine and Health Care.
Includes bibliographical references.
ISBN 0 471 92634 5
1. Medical ethics—Congresses. 2. Medical care—Decision making—Congresses. I. Jensen, Uffe Juul. II. Mooney, Gavin H. III. European Society for Philosophy of Medicine and Health Care.
[DNLM: 1. Decision Making—congresses. 2. Delivery of Health Care—congresses. 3. Philosophy, Medical—congresses. W 84.1 C4565 1988]
R724.C44 1990
174'.2—dc20
DLC
for Library of Congress 89-70700
CIP

British Library Cataloguing in Publication Data
Changing values in medical and health care decision making.
1. Medicine. Decision making
I. Jensen, U. J. (Uffe Juul) II. Mooney, Gavin, *1943–*
610

ISBN 0 471 92634 5

Phototypeset by Dobbie Typesetting Limited, Plymouth, Devon

Contents

Contributors

TAMAS ANGELUS, PhD, *Institute of Social Medicine and History of Medicine, Semmelweis University of Medicine, Hungary*

INGER BRØDSGAARD, MD, *Aarhus University, Denmark*

HENK TEN HAVE, *Physician and Philosopher, Professor, Department of Health Care Ethics and Philosophy, University of Limburg, The Netherlands*

MATTI HAKAMA, ScD, *Epidemiologist, Tampere University Central Hospital, Finland*

KAIJA HOLLI, MD, *Oncologist, Tampere University Central Hospital, Finland*

UFFE JUUL JENSEN, PhD, *Professor of Philosophy, Aarhus University, Denmark*

GERRIT KIMSMA, *General Practitioner and Philosopher, Westzaan, The Netherlands*

HELGE KJERSEM, MD, *State Serum Institute, Copenhagen, Denmark*

PER-ERIK LISS, BA, *Department of Health and Society, Linköping University, Sweden*

ERICH H. LOEWY, MD, *Associate Professor of Medicine, University of Illinois College of Medicine at Peoria, and Associate Professor of Humanities (Ethics) University of Illinois College of Medicine, Peoria, USA*

GAVIN MOONEY, MA, *Professor of Health Economics, University of Copenhagen, Denmark*

ROD MOORE, DDS, MA, *Royal College of Dentistry, Aarhus, Denmark*

LENNART NORDENFELT, PhD, *Professor, Department of Health and Society, Linköping University, Sweden*

KENNETH MCKENZIE NORRIE, LLB, DLP, PhD, *Lecturer in Law, University of Aberdeen, Scotland*

ROEL OTTEN, Drs, *Research Assistant, Department of Philosophy, University of Limburg, The Netherlands*

P. J. THUNG, MD, *Physician, Psychiatric Hospital, 'Endegeest', Oegstgeest, The Netherlands*

R. J. VERKES, MD, *Professor, Department 'METAMEDICA', Medical Faculty, University of Leiden, The Netherlands*

G. L. WACKERS, MD, *Department of Health Care Ethics and Philosophy, University of Limburg, The Netherlands*

GUY WIDDERSHOVEN, PhD, *Associate Professor, Department of Health Care Ethics and Philosophy, University of Limburg, The Netherlands*

INEKE WIDDERSHOVEN-HEERDING, PhD, *Lecturer, Open University, The Netherlands*

Foreword

This book originated in an international conference on values in medical decision making held at the University of Aarhus, Denmark, in June 1988. This was the second conference of the European Society for Philosophy of Medicine and Health Care (ESPMH), founded in Maastricht, The Netherlands, in 1987. ESPMH aims at promoting philosophy of medicine and health care in a wide sense and at stimulating contacts between European scholars in this field. It is therefore most gratifying when an ESPMH conference ultimately results in a publication reaching out to a wider public. Professors Jensen of Aarhus and Mooney of Copenhagen, who jointly had the lead in organizing the Aarhus conference, have now succeeded in collating a number of stimulating papers dealing with 'values' in relation to medicine. ESPMH is very appreciative of their energy and resourcefulness in making a success of both the conference and the book.

This volume is intended to be part of a series of similar publications reflecting the activities of ESPMH in furthering the development of medical philosophy in Europe.

P. J. Thung
ESPMH President 1987–1989
Leiden, Summer 1989

1

Changing Values: Autonomy and Paternalism in Medicine and Health Care

Uffe Juul Jensen, PhD and Gavin Mooney, MA

1. INTRODUCTION

In recent years there has been a general slowing down in the rate of growth of expenditure on health care in the majority of the Organization for Economic Co-operation and Development (OECD) industrialised countries (OECD, 1987). While there remain substantial differences in the level of spending in different countries, most of the decision makers in the health care systems appear to be becoming much more aware of the fact that resources for health care are not unlimited.

This fact is not new. It is only the extent of the awareness that is new. More and more there are discussions and debate about the advantages and disadvantages of different financing systems; about the concept of efficiency; about the role of the medical profession vis-à-vis the patient, vis-à-vis the government, vis-à-vis the insurance companies, vis-à-vis society; about the role of equity in health care; about the pace of technological development and societies' abilities to afford the new technologies; and how to appraise not just new but also old technologies.

The debate and discussions are real. But do they lead to any change? There have been some changes with respect to the organisation of health care. Health maintenance organisations (HMOs) and diagnostic related groups (DRGs) are spreading in the United States and indeed beyond. The United Kingdom government, as we write, is about to publish a major review of the National Health Service. The 'threat' of the growing costs of care of the elderly has provoked several governments to institute changes and experiments to contain costs. Concern that the public purse cannot cope

Changing Values in Medical and Health Care Decision Making
Edited by U. J. Jensen and G. Mooney

has pushed the Danish government to consider major increases in patient payments.

There is organisational change afoot. What is less clear is how fundamental it is and how far-reaching it will be. It is not just that aspects of supply and demand are changing; so is the ability to measure the output of our health care industry. As the systems change, as budgets tighten, as output is measured, as efficiency becomes an accepted goal in health care, it is relevant to consider what is happening to the values that underpin our institutions both of health care and of medicine.

This book examines changing values in medicine and in health care. Its starting point was a conference of the European Society for Philosophy of Medicine and Health Care in Århus in June 1988. Some of the papers in this volume were presented in another form at that meeting but have since been rewritten. Others have been specially invited. The emphasis in all is on change.

The authors come from several different backgrounds and countries. No attempt has been made to select them however on any basis other than the fact that their paper 'fitted'. (Some did not and were therefore not accepted.) However seeing the final product we believe as editors that through a little cajoling and a lot of good luck and good will we have a series of readings on the theme of the book which, despite the different national and disciplinary perspectives, constitutes a rounded entity. We hope you as reader will agree.

In this opening chapter we emphasise one theme: given the pressure of increased awareness of limited resources in health care, what can we say about the values underlying medicine and health care as we enter the decade leading to the year 2000? Our task, a seemingly simple one, has been complicated (but by less than we expected!) by the different perspectives of the editors—Uffe a philosopher and Gavin an economist. That has made for an exciting journey in the process of the writing of this chapter. But we are well aware that the many joins may very readily be seen. We hope these are viewed by the reader as legitimate but at the same time that they do not disturb the flow of ideas too much.

We have not rounded off this introductory chapter in a neat tightly packaged way. It was never our intention to do so, which is fortunate because now we see where we have been we are not quite clear where we would go to achieve that tightly packaged article. Perhaps it will emerge through the other authors. We will attempt at least to draw the various strands together in the concluding chapter.

It is worth mentioning the process involved in this writing. We proposed the theme for the book and invited potential authors to submit synopses of papers. We then selected from amongst these and commented on those selected to try to help the authors to understand better how their offering might fit in the book as a whole. A draft of this chapter was then circulated to all authors who thereafter completed first drafts of their chapters. We as editors commented on all draft chapters, the authors revised their work and we wrote the final chapter.

Beyond this introduction we have concentrated on what we believe is crucial in the context of values to health care at present, to this book and to our chapter: the issue of autonomy, partly vis-à-vis paternalism, but also as an entity in itself and how best it can be defined. Thereafter we have attempted to relate this largely conceptual discussion to some practical issues of health care resource allocation.

In the final section we list a few questions in this context that we do not answer at this point. Rather we hope that our fellow authors may pick up on some of them—allowing us to come back to them in a more informed way than we could at present in the concluding chapter of the book.

2. VALUES IN HEALTH CARE

2.1. From paternalism to autonomy

Basic values have been changing recently in health care. For centuries or even millennia paternalism or the role of the expert has moulded the key relationship in health care—that between doctor and patient.

Now autonomy is espoused as the basic value for the modern health care system. Surprisingly too, such espousal appears almost universal: doctors, other professional groups, patients and politicians—all are apparently advocating autonomy as the ethical basis of modern health care.

There are many reasons for this change in values. Traditional forms of paternalism and expert attitudes have been associated with (or justified by reference to) specific ideals of medical thinking and a specific concept of disease. These have had an influence on medical thinking which has endured from antiquity almost until today and which only recently has come under fire. Health care problems have always been defined with reference to particular diseases. In turn diseases have been interpreted as, in principle, well defined entities, the essence of which would in the long run be revealed by medical thinking and science. This view was linked to another basic idea: that of specific treatment according to which there is, in principle, one specific cure or treatment (or preventive strategy) for any disease.

These classical ideals were associated with the foundationalist epistemology and philosophy of science which came to dominate modern philosophy from the 17th century onwards. Experimental science would (it was claimed) in the long run present us with absolutely true explanations of the phenomena of nature (including human diseases), and thereby science would provide the opportunity to control nature—and society—completely.

Foundationalist philosophy provided the natural sciences with an extraordinary legitimisation of power and authority at the expense of the power and authority of the Church or the state and their institutions. So Bacon's famous phrase 'knowledge is power' not only expresses the basic insight that knowledge extends our possibilities of action and thereby our power over nature. It is also an expression of the ideology of modern society that scientific knowledge (and not for example being called by God) justifies authority in the context of society and its problems.

In the second part of this century foundationalism has generally been rejected as a myth and as an ideology used in glorifying particular scientific contributions, having only relative validity rather than expressing a valid analysis of the content and functioning of scientific knowledge.

It is interesting, however, that in the same period when foundationalism was abandoned in epistemology and philosophy of science, it continued to be the espoused philosophy of biomedical science. Foundationalist ideas are still used in attempts to legitimise the supreme status of biomedical research in health care. This is especially true for those biomedical specialties which try to explain the biological mechanisms lying behind common diseases (such as cancer) or which use advanced diagnostic technologies (such as scanners) in attempts to make exact and objective criteria for the diagnosis of disease. In this way, foundationalist ideas still play a role in the continuing fight to get as large a share as possible of scarce resources.

This essentially ideological stance is perhaps one of the reasons why foundationalism is now under heavy fire. Other professional groups, both within and outside health care, do not willingly accept that the biomedical specialties (which have continued to attempt to legitimise their authority by the promulgation of philosophical myths) have first priority when scarce resources are being allocated. It is, correctly, claimed that many different kinds of experience and knowledge and different kinds of research and practice can and should be involved in improving the quality of health care. It is claimed that psychological and sociological knowledge, together with humanistic insights, should play a much more central role in health care. And as these ideas of 'absoluteness' on which foundationalism is based simply do not make sense within these other scientific fields, the biomedical specialties have had difficulties in keeping alive the old idea (and ideal) of the omnipotent doctor (Jensen, 1987).

At the same time patients and patient organisations are contributing to the undermining of the concept of absolute authority. This is partly as a result of the more critical attitude to experts which has developed in most western societies over the last 20 to 30 years. It is also in part a result of frustration because of unfulfilled promises from biomedical specialties (e.g. in cancer research). This frustration has sometimes developed into distrust towards scientific medicine and into growing interest in various kinds of holistic medicine which advocate both research and therapeutic strategies radically different from that research and therapy developed in scientific medicine.

2.2. Varieties of autonomy

Thus paternalism and what might be termed the arrogance of the expert are under fire. Autonomy has become the value espoused in the eighties and will probably remain so in the nineties. It is however difficult to assess the accompanying change which has taken place and to predict its probable consequences for the health care system. Closer scrutiny reveals that it is not just one particular value, autonomy, that is at play. Behind the widespread, almost unanimous, appeal to autonomy at least three different values (related to different ethical positions) are present and being expressed.

In the face of this one might be inclined to draw the conclusion that there is nothing to discuss and analyse here. It might be claimed that autonomy is purely an ideological term used by different persons or groups just to express their private interests and attitudes with the result that there are no conceptual matters present which can be handled by philosophical and scientific tools.

This, however, is to rush to a conclusion based on a superficial understanding of values and value statements. Value statements are not just expressions of personal feelings or attitudes. They are, as is the case for any other use of words, expressed within a common language, used within a specific set of human circumstances. A value-laden term such as autonomy is, as with any other term or expression, used and taught in concrete situations. Consequently its meaning can be specified by looking for ideal or prototypical situations in which to apply the term in question.

The varieties of autonomy at play in the modern health care system can be accounted for by analysing, from the standpoint of various different principles of autonomy, the different contexts within which autonomy is assumed to occur. In one sense, as based on deontological ethics, autonomy is conceived of as a basic right (to be respected by both the doctor and other professionals). Autonomy in this context is said to obtain when an individual, presented with adequate information about his or her situation, makes his or her own personal choice, free from any external coercion or interference (Engelhardt, 1986, 1988). Such autonomy is today advocated by many members of the medical profession. However it has a broader ideological appeal. It has not only implications for the relationship between therapist and patient but also appears to have important consequences for health care policy (as we discuss later).

Autonomy, as advocated in a different form, is closely associated with ethical relativism. Autonomy here is claimed to be attained in a social context when differences in human attitudes and values are respected. Self-determination is not, as is the case with deontologists, conceived of as being indigenous to man. According to this relativistic position, there are no absolute rights at all (or rather it makes no sense to speak of innate rights). The claim of autonomy is then not a positive claim. It is, rather, negative, to the effect that there are no absolute standards with regard to what constitutes a good human life, human dignity, etc. It follows that individual attitudes (and especially differences in attitudes) have to be taken into account when the quality of a person's life is being measured or when, for example, it has to be decided if prolongation of life or quality of life should be the dominant value on which decisions should be made on which treatment to give to which individual.

There is a third type of autonomy. According to this concept, which finds expression in the World Health Organization (WHO) programme *Health for all by the year 2000* (WHO, 1983), autonomy is not a power or resource, something which the individual person has and which he or she has a basic duty to use. Nor is it just a claim to the effect that values are our private individual creations. Rather autonomy is conceived as an end, but one which can only be realised under specific social conditions. It is an ideal situation where we act as responsible persons in relation to our own lives and to those of others. Further, autonomy is not something which arises just because the necessary external conditions are provided by society. It is a complex way of behaving which has to be acquired, which the individual has to learn (WHO, 1983).

This conception of autonomy is associated with the ethical principle of solidarity according to which we are social beings dependent upon each other but having the possibility of compensating for or overcoming our weakness through mutual support. This form of autonomy should be distinguished from the deontological and relativist ethics embodied in the first and second kinds of autonomy, both of which express individualistic conceptions of man.

3. AUTONOMY AS A BASIC RIGHT AND DUTY (DEONTOLOGICAL AUTONOMY)

This form of autonomy is advocated in a number of situations involving ethical controversy in modern health care. The patient has a *right*, it is claimed, to decide for himself or herself between various therapeutic strategies, or to decide if he or she wants any treatment at all. Autonomy is espoused as a defence against traditional paternalism.

For example, the genetic counsellor should provide information as clearly and as neutrally as possible about the genetic test, the risk of provoking an abortion by carrying out the test, the result of the test, etc., but it is the pregnant woman (perhaps with her partner) who should decide if the test is to be carried out and if she, having been informed of abnormal findings, wants an abortion. However it is relevant to ask how free and autonomous the woman is at the moment of choice. What of the woman who, having wanted a baby for years, now at the age of 38 and finally having become pregnant, is told that in undergoing the test there is a risk of provoking an abortion, a risk which is equal to that of finding some serious genetic abnormality? If the woman asks the counsellor to assist her in making the difficult choices, the counsellor will, if he/she acts in the light of the deontological principle of autonomy, refuse. The woman should make her own decision. Some might question if the woman is genuinely free in such a situation of emotional distress but on the basis of the principle as stated, she is free. If she is well informed about the various possibilities of action and if no one is forcing her to choose one thing rather than another, then she is by definition in a position to act autonomously.

Critics of the deontological conception of autonomy will argue that real freedom of choice has pre-conditions other than just the absence of physical coercion. Doctors and other professionals who now widely adopt this notion of autonomy are criticised for avoiding their professional duty and responsibility.

It is not surprising that deontological autonomy appeals to patients and patient organisations, who are critical of traditional forms of paternalism. But why is this form of autonomy now widely espoused by medical doctors, who traditionally acted paternalistically? And why is it that such autonomy has become a central value in the broader ideological discussion surrounding changes in health care systems?

In practice, it is not surprising that doctors, who are still in a position of power in most health care systems, are willing to accept this principle. They can subscribe to the principle without running any serious risk of undermining their own power base, so long as the more basic structure of the health care system and the organisation and functioning of its institutions are not challenged. Various organisational conditions will continue to constrain the patients' possibilities for choice and for action and such constraints can easily be veiled behind the advocacy of patients' rights.

This principle of autonomy may also seem attractive to doctors in a climate in which rationing of health care is indicated explicitly and in a situation where many politicians, planners, philosophers and others are questioning whether doctors should play any role at all in the process of rationing health care.

According to the principle of autonomy as discussed here, the introduction of new therapeutic strategies is justified to the extent that these help to extend the patients' range of choice (and action). But if it is agreed that it is impossible to continue indefinitely to develop and make available new therapeutic strategies, how then should health care be rationed according to the principle of deontological autonomy?

The prime strategy for rationing health care that emerges from this principle of autonomy is that of the private market. It is the neoclassical market model that supports this form of autonomy or more accurately perhaps, it is on this principle of autonomy that the free market is based (Mishan, 1981). The informed rational consumer chooses on the demand side of the market and independently on the supply side, through the relevant price signals provided in the market, the producers respond to try to achieve an efficient solution to the rationing process. It is the neoclassical economist's 'consumer sovereignty'—where consumers have no choice whether they want to be sovereign or not (McGuire *et al.*, 1988).

Even patient payments in public health care may have an element of this form of autonomy present if it is the case that such payments are aimed at informing patient choice and at placing more responsibility on the patient to do his or her own choosing. Thus the concern which is often expressed to avoid or at least to contain 'moral hazard' (the idea that subsidising health care may result not only in 'overconsumption' of health services but in individuals not taking adequate care of their own health; Pauly, 1968) may well be born of the desire to pursue this form of patient autonomy in health care decision making.

4. RELATIVISTIC AUTONOMY

According to deontological autonomy, individuals have to carry the burden of freedom and autonomy even if this leads to personal dissatisfaction or unhappiness. The principle of deontological autonomy expresses an ideal of human dignity which is quite incompatible with ideas of quality of life as they are usually presented in modern health care. Deontological autonomy implies that there is one final and absolute answer to the question of what a human life of quality is. It is a life where we are free to act responsibly without taking into account our personal inclinations and attitudes as individuals as to whether we want to act in this way.

Deontological autonomy can be clearly contrasted with another conception of autonomy which is widely advocated in modern health care and indeed in modern society in general. Here the appeal to autonomy is to the effect that each individual person has a right to adopt his or her own attitudes and preferences (values) and that there is no such thing as an absolute value-yardstick. Therefore the individual person's own needs and preferences should be taken into account and respected by a health care system espousing this form of autonomy as its basic ethical principle.

Such relativistic autonomy not only runs counter to deontological autonomy due to the radically different ethical underpinnings of each. The two kinds of autonomy also have significantly different implications regarding the concrete question: How should the health care system be organised to respect the autonomy of the patient?

According to deontological autonomy the basic condition for realisation of autonomy is, as pointed out above, that the patient is well informed about the various therapeutic strategies which might possibly be used in his or her case.

The situation is more complicated from the standpoint of relativistic autonomy. The patient makes his or her choice to have his or her preferences and needs satisfied. The system should accept that and not force the patient to adopt values which are not his or her own.

This does not, however, imply that professional assistance is superfluous. Since there are no absolute yardsticks of value, we are within our rights to insist on our own values and to try to have them realised. Often however we are confused about our personal preferences, needs and values. The nature of the transaction in health care between patient and doctor is such that the doctor acts as an informing agent on behalf of the often ignorant, insecure and potentially irrational patient/consumer (Arrow, 1963). We may be inclined to act in a way which, in the long run, will lead to dissatisfaction and unhappiness. So professionals (psychologists, sociologists, economists and others) who through their research can present justified assumptions about ways of handling contradictory preferences, of assessing harmful consequences of choices which are immediately attractive, etc. have an important role to play in a health care system which accepts the principle of relativistic autonomy.

In this way the asymmetry of information between patient and doctor results in the patient seeking to have the doctor acting on his or her behalf not just in supplying care but also in assisting in making demands which are in the patient's interests. This is the so-called 'agency relationship' (Evans, 1984) which is a central concept in much of today's economic deliberations in health care.

It is thus not surprising that relativistic autonomy has been widely espoused by non-medical professionals (and by general practitioners and psychiatrists), while deontological autonomy remains attractive to medical specialists. This is perhaps inevitable when the latter group's power and authority in the health care system have, in recent years, been questioned by the former group.

The difference between the principle of deontological autonomy and that of relativistic autonomy can be further illuminated by considering the implications of each concerning how health care is rationed. Stated boldly, deontologial autonomy with its emphasis on an informed, rational patient able, willing and indeed having to act as the sovereign consumer points to a market system of health care. It is the neoclassical man who decides. The invisible hand of Adam Smith—the influence of market prices ensuring efficiency—dominates and regulation is non-existent or minimal. Suppliers in aggregate and consumers in aggregate meet in the market place as equals.

It is more difficult to state precisely what the implications are for rationing health care stemming from the principle of relativistic autonomy. It could be a public health care system but that is unlikely since, according to the principle of relativistic autonomy, no one has the scientific or moral authority to formulate the goals of health care. Normally public health care systems are public at least in part because of recognition of a political authority to set goals. Indeed sceptics might argue that relativistic autonomy, allowing both patients and citizens their own values and preferences, leads to anarchy and makes impossible any kind of societal or political planning. If this is true, then relativistic autonomy could also pave the way for a private market in health care.

The reality would seem to lie somewhere in between, with what is best described as a heavily regulated market for health care, i.e. regulated by government and/or other public agencies. There is an asymmetry of information in the health care market which suggests that deontological autonomy, which requires a fully informed consumer/patient, does not apply in practice.

However the individualism underpinning relativistic autonomy—the rights of individuals to have different preferences—is in our view best seen in private market terms, albeit some distance from the 'perfect' neoclassical market we discussed before. In the regulated private insurance world which is such a common feature of so many western nations' health care systems, the individual's preferences still count but the supply side of the market is constrained because of the need for an agent to act on the patient's behalf. Thus the key principle of relativistic autonomy in health care is enshrined in the notions of freedom of choice of the patient but accepting now that the patient may well need help from the doctor to decide what his or her preferences are. It is with this form of autonomy that the exercise of clinical freedom—present in all forms of health care rationing—is most crucial as it both accepts that the patient cannot be deontologically autonomous and at the same time attempts to promote the individual patient's own preferences (as seen through the eyes of the doctor) as well as possible. (It may be worth emphasising here that when clinical freedom is defined as 'doing what is best for the patient' ideally this is to be interpreted as what the patient would judge was best were he/she fully informed, prudent and rational.)

The advocate of relativistic autonomy may respond that the view that values are personal does not imply that the organisation of social life is impossible. It appears that we often share values with other people. And the political institutions of liberal democracy are our very efficient means of aggregating the individual, personal values of the citizens. We express our values when voting at democratic elections. Politicians and parties then represent our values and try as far as possible to have the shared values of their voters realised in laws and policies generally.

In democratic negotiations over laws and policy, doctors and other professional groups have no role to play. The doctor may influence the political process by taking part in the public debate, by joining a party, etc., but as a doctor he or she has no special right to influence health policy. On the contrary, democratic society, once it accepts the principle of relativistic autonomy, should take all necessary precautions to exclude 'experts' such as doctors from influencing health policy.

Experts will, of course, still have roles to play in the political process, for example in accounting for their expertise in an objective and neutral way, illuminating the benefits as well as the costs and risks in using their professional knowledge and techniques in a particular field. But recognising that resources are scarce, health policy or policy in any other field should be based on more general, primarily social and economic considerations, rather than on the considerations of specialists trained within narrow fields.

5. SOCIAL AUTONOMY

The principle of social autonomy implies a rejection of the individualism presupposed by deontological autonomy and relativistic autonomy. According to this principle it makes no sense to claim either that we are autonomous beings and that society ought simply to protect our right to act in accordance with this innate gift or that the values expressed in our preferences or choices are our personal creations. Values are common, they are embodied in concrete exemplars of ideal patterns of action which regulate any human community. Our whole moral language—and our ethical concepts of rights and obligations—are acquired in social contexts, as ways of characterising and assessing relationships of power and dependence between individuals.

If we were free floating atoms or Robinson Crusoes there would be no room for ethics. Today, from birth, we are embedded in relationships of dependence and power. Here one of the most basic human experiences is that weaknesses in the form of illnesses, social problems, educational needs, etc., weaknesses which for a shorter or longer time may undermine our autonomy, can be compensated for or overcome by support from our fellow-beings who have it in their power to support us and liberate us from our weakness. In these ordinary experiences the most basic principle of ethics of ordinary life is embedded.

We acquire the principle of interpersonal responsibility in our day-to-day lives and in our intercourse with other individuals. But where in the variety of types of human interaction do we find models of responsible behaviour? Is it possible to find some basis for our ordinary activities around which our language for describing human behaviour as being more or less responsible develops? To locate this, a first important step is to characterise the relationship which seems to obtain between individuals or groups in any kind of human community. At a given time a person, B, is in the power of some other person, A, in the sense that A can cause B to do things he would not have done otherwise. Parents have this kind of power over their children, professionals over their clients and patients.

In our everyday understanding there is a distinction between the legitimate, morally responsible, and the illegitimate, morally irresponsible, use of power. Our model for morally responsible use of power can be summed up as follows: when A causes B to do something which he would not have done otherwise, then A is acting morally responsibly if his actions towards B aim at or contribute to making B independent of the power of A, or of others having a similar power. To describe this model-activity in ordinary terms, we are acting morally responsibly towards other individuals or groups who in a particular context are weaker than us, if we try to act from their point of view, and support them. This activity, assumed to be the model-activity communal life, is not confined to priests or philosophers. It can be summed up as the basic moral principle of responsibility for the weak. Due to the existence of such model-activities in our everyday life, ordinary people (and not only experts in theology, ethics or moral psychology) possess, and are able to use, a language of morals for commenting on past and future actions, often to create excuses for actions which we recognise as violating the basic moral principle.

The moral principle prescribing responsibility for the weaknesses of others is to be explained by reference to the basic constraint of human communal life. We are involved in relationships characterised by dependence and power; we are not independent and self-sufficient individuals (Churchill, 1987; Jensen, 1987).

We have a well founded knowledge to the effect that many kinds of weakness and dependence (in particular social problems and health problems) are due to our way of organising society and to environmental and working conditions. These cannot be changed by individuals and, according to the principle of social autonomy, those having the power necessary for fighting the weakness and vulnerability of particular groups have a responsibility to support the weak groups in society. Further, society and its political authorities have a responsibility to develop a policy for organising support for such a policy. This principle of solidarity or social autonomy is embodied in the WHO programme *Health for all by the year 2000*, being expressed in aims to secure justice or equity in health care. Such a principle not only provides a justification for the existence of a public health care system; it also provides us with a basic ethical principle for rationing health care.

It is a political, social (or group) solution for the protection of those who are ill. It is not charity because although some are 'weaker' than others in the sense that they either are more ill or are at greater risk, all are at risk to some extent. Consequently the protection of the weak means the protection of us all.

But it is not just in the sense of being ill or at risk of being ill that we as individuals are weak. Given the nature of the health care sector as a supplier we are weak as individual consumers. Health care as a social institution suffers from the same problem as medicine at an individual patient level: the asymmetry of information. However, while in both situations the patient and the citizen often seek an agent to assist them with information and the decision making process, it is less clear at the social institution level who the agent should be.

Part of the role of a public health care system is for the public authorities to act as the citizen's agent in planning, priority setting and controlling health care. But while such sentiments or values may be common to many societies, the solution of a public health care system is only tenable in circumstances where there is a sufficient degree of solidarity—or homogeneity of values—in the society to allow social autonomy to be the dominating value.

Another view based on social autonomy is put forward by Margolis (1982), as adapted by one of the authors (Mooney, 1986). Margolis argues that each individual has two utility functions as opposed to the one normally attributed to individuals by economic theorists. One utility function is of a more or less normal type and is concerned with the utility or satisfaction the consumer derives from the consumption of goods and services. (This is in utilitarian terms essentially a consequentialist view of the world where only consequences—here goods and services—have utility bearing characteristics.) Margolis suggests that there is also utility in 'participation' or what he calls doing our fair share, i.e. that individuals want to 'do their bit' for some group, community or society. The utility to the individual here is obtained from the doing: not from the consequences of the doing.

GHM has argued previously (Mooney, 1986) that health care is a particularly important area for the application of this theory, primarily because we are all to some extent concerned with the need of all to have access to health care services. This makes the justice and distributional aspects important. But the various key features of health care—uncertainty, irrationality, unpredictability, ignorance—also makes us aware that we are weak as consumers. Where we are confident that others share our values, then we may seek a common solution: the public ownership and supply of health care services.

In this system there is some overlap with relativistic autonomy since some attempt is made to allow individuals' different preferences to be retained. But there is more standardisation which pushes towards common values.

It is under such a system however that the traditional deontological autonomy of the medical profession becomes most problematical and some of the constraints on the freedom of the profession, already present in the regulated private market, become tightened under public health care and hence still more problematical. Who decides for health services on objectives and priorities? The answer in principle under social autonomy is clear. It is the public authorities on behalf of the citizenry. Yet clinical freedom is maintained and objectives and priorities at a clinical level remain very much the province of the doctors. There is an inevitable tension in the middle.

It is possible to see substantial variations in the organisation and financing of health services across different countries. It is also clearly possible to see different value systems in different countries—Eastern Europe; Scandinavia; the United Kingdom; the United States; Mediterranean Europe, and so on. To some extent—but we would not want to exaggerate it— there is some relationship between the nature of the society and the nature of health care. Thus it comes as no great surprise that Scandinavia with its social democratic traditions has largely public, decentralised health care systems; nor that the more individualistically minded United States remains, despite heavy regulation, more market orientated in its health care than most other countries.

6. SOME ISSUES

It follows that one of the key value issues in health care today is: Who holds the property rights over which decisions? As the mix of the different forms of autonomy changes over time so, in our view, does the distribution of these property rights. Who decides what? Who should decide,what? How best should health care be organised in the future to reflect changing values? Who shall live and who shall die? And who has the right to decide?

What are the objectives of health care? of medicine? Are they the same? changing? What is the role of the medical doctor in health care policy? What do patients want from their doctors? What do citizens want from their health care systems?

Where do we sit on the spectrum from deontological autonomy, through relativistic and social autonomy to paternalism? Where should we sit? And does it matter in which country the question is posed? How do values affect the concept of need for health care? Can we measure need? Can we measure health—given that that fundamental concept is itself value-laden? As concepts of autonomy change how do ethics and ethical codes react?

As resource constraints bite how do the organisational structures of health care change? Do values change?

The choices facing health services today are choices about values and are dictated by values. Yet the discussion of values in medicine and health care—and of the implications of the *changes* in values—has been muted. There is a need for more debate and in the pages that follow our fellow contributors to this volume tackle some of the key issues. In the final chapter we attempt to draw some strands together when considering future values in health care.

REFERENCES

Arrow, K. J. (1963) Uncertainty and the welfare economics of medical care. *American Economics Review* **53**, 941–73.

Churchill, L. R. (1987) *Rationing Health Care in America.* University of Notre Dame Press, Notre Dame.

Engelhardt, H. T. (1986) *The Foundation of Bio-ethics.* Oxford University Press, New York.

Engelhardt, H. T. (1988) Morality for the medical-industrial complex. *New England Journal of Medicine* **16**, 1086–89.

Evans, R. G. (1984) *Strained Mercy.* Butterworth, Toronto.

Jensen, U. J. (1987) *Practice and Progress. A Theory of Modern Health Care Systems.* Blackwell Scientific Publications, Oxford.

Margolis, H. (1982) *Selfishness, Altruism and Rationality.* Cambridge University Press, Cambridge.

McGuire, A., Henderson, J. and Mooney, G. (1988) *The Economics of Health Care.* Routledge and Kegan Paul, London.

Mishan, E. J. (1981) *Cost Benefit Analysis.* Allen and Unwin, London.

Mooney, G. H. (1986) *Economics, Medicine and Health Care.* Wheatsheaf, Brighton.

OECD (1987) *Financing and Delivering Health Care.* OECD, Paris.

Pauly, M. V. (1968) The economics of moral hazard: a comment. *American Economics Review* **57**, 231–7.

WHO (1983) *Targets in Support of the Regional Strategy for Health for All 2000.* WHO/EURO, Copenhagen.

2

Commodities, Needs and Health Care: A Communal Perspective

Erich H. Loewy, MD

This chapter examines the concept of needs. Basic needs are divided into basic biologically determined 'first order' and into basic socially determined 'second order' necessities. It is argued that health care (as well as education) are basic second order necessities. Various ways of looking at community structure, and the ideas of justice which flow from such views, are examined. Unless one accepts what I argue to be a flawed concept of a starkly minimalist community (in which no moral obligation other than mutual non-harm is recognized), a more beneficent model emerges.

If one accepts a minimalist community, in which freedom and autonomy are absolutes, no obligations to provide any sort of needs exist. On the other hand, if one accepts at least minimal beneficence as a moral obligation, it is argued that one must assure at least basic first order necessities to all members before allowing opulent luxuries to others. Communities which assure nothing beyond this, however, are fated to develop an ever-enlarging class of the disadvantaged and eventually succumb to violence. Democracy in such communities is a cynical mockery. Communities which attempt to provide second order necessities to all, prior to allowing some the enjoyment of opulent luxuries, provide a more fertile ground for democracy, evolution and growth.

Changing Values in Medical and Health Care Decision Making
Edited by U. J. Jensen and G. Mooney

1. INTRODUCTION

One can look at health care and the right to health care in a variety of ways. On the one hand, one can consider health care to be a commodity like any other commodity and, therefore, to be traded in the market place like TV sets, theatre tickets, or washing machines. On the other hand, one can hold that health care is somehow different and that because of that difference it is a commodity which all members of a just community, by virtue of being members of such a community, deserve. Unless one claims that all commodities (even TV sets, theatre tickets or washing machines) should be distributed in an absolutely equal fashion to all members of the community, one needs to justify why it is that health care and certain other things are different from other commodities and, furthermore, different enough to warrant special attention. Special attention does not necessarily imply that a two-tiered system of health care is not possible; it does suggest that basic health care, as we shall define it, has moral standing a good deal different from TV sets, theatre tickets or washing machines. If one finds that health care does have special standing among other commodities (if, for example, one holds that it is a basic need in modern societies), one still may hold either that communities do or that they do not have an intrinsic obligation to see to it that all members of the community have at least a decent minimum of their basic needs met. Which stand one then takes depends upon whether one thinks that basic health care is or is not vital to modern life, and on the way one looks at community and, therefore, at the way one conceives of justice.

In this paper I want to examine:

1. the notion of needs;
2. health care as a basic need;
3. different ways of looking at the structure of community and, therefore, different ways of conceiving of justice;
4. I want to offer a brief argument that in the modern world, communities have an obligation to see to it that the basic needs of all members are met before allowing some to have exorbitant luxuries.

2. THE NOTION OF NEEDS

The concept of needs is often appealed to. Yet unless one defines what a need is and what it is not rather carefully, such appeals become mere slogans. A need, in ordinary language, can be almost anything from a passing fancy to a vital condition of my existence. A 'need' (like an 'ought' in a hypothetical) is the means necessary to the attainment of a given goal. I need to look into a shop-window to satisfy my curiosity as to what it contains, I need air in order to live; both are 'needs'. Using the language of needs indicates only that the indicated 'need' is required in order to attain a given goal: it is the goal, and the likelihood that the means can attain the goal, which determines the importance of the need, not the fact that something is or is not a need. Needs, furthermore, while they may be the necessary condition for attaining a given end may not, by themselves, be a sufficient condition. Other conditions may have to be met. To continue my existence, I need food, water, shelter and many more things. Any one of these describes a 'need'; satisfying any one of these, however, is not a sufficient condition for continuing my existence.

Basic needs, as I will define them, are basic because unless such needs are met biosocial existence is either impossible or hopelessly impoverished. Needs which do not serve such biologically or socially defined ends are not basic needs: TV sets, theatre tickets or washing machines in our particular society, even if not, perhaps, in all conceivable societies, would be examples. In turn, I will divide such basic needs into 'first order' and 'second order necessities'.

By 'first order necessities' I shall mean those things needed to sustain normal, natural biological life. Food, water, clothing and shelter are examples. Such needs are biologically conditioned: they form the necessary underpinnings of normal life. First order necessities are universal needs, common and necessary to all humans no matter when or where. They are what makes biological existence possible; without them, and inevitably, we die.

On the other hand, I shall consider basic 'second order necessities' to be those things needed to sustain an acceptable existence in a given social context. I shall argue that in modern, industrialized societies, education and health care are basic second order necessities. Second order needs vary; they are not fixed and not necessarily defined by biology as are first order needs, but rather such needs are defined by the particular social condition in which such a biological organism finds itself. What is and what is not a second order need is ultimately determined by the community.

Just because something is a basic need, however, does not entail that communities have an obligation to meet such needs. Individual needs, no matter whether defined individually or by the community, are, after all, the needs of an individual and may well, therefore, be the responsibility of the individual. But things are not that simple: as Churchill (1987) has pointed out, while needs are individual needs, they are socially defined and validated. Some feel that communities by their very definition and constitution have obligations to try to meet at least a decent minimum of basic needs. Others, however, feel that while the community and the individuals within it may well have an obligation not to harm their fellows by standing in the way of their needs, no obligation to facilitate such needs exists.

3. HEALTH CARE AS A BASIC NEED

I shall argue that health care is a basic second order necessity. To say that it is a first order, biologically determined, necessity implies that without health care people will not be able to exist. While this may be the case for some persons and for some persons at some time in their lives, normal, natural life does not invariably require health care to sustain it. Normal, natural life invariably requires food, water, and shelter. In that sense, health care is not quite the same. An infant can grow into mature adulthood and healthy old age and ultimately die in the natural order of things without ever needing to be sustained by medical care; the same cannot be said of food, water or shelter.

In the vitalist presumption, life itself (at least human life) is a 'good' worth pursuing at all costs. Those who cling to this point of view see the value of life as self-justifying: life (or at least human life) is of value because it lives. Such a position, of course, entails sustaining every vestige of life (or, at least, of human life) come what may. Content may or may not be important: but it is, at any rate, a secondary consideration. Few would hold such an extreme point of view. Those who do not share such a point of view consider life to be of value as the necessary condition for experience or, put in a different way, to be of value because of the biography that such a life underwrites (Rachels, 1986; Loewy, 1987a). Such a point of view will focus on the nature of the experience rather than merely on the biological condition of life itself.

Viewing life as the necessary condition for experience and sustaining life for that reason implies a healthy respect for social conditions. Our experiences are inevitably biosocial. Meeting first order necessities provides a necessary but hardly a sufficient condition: the necessary conditions for life itself to continue (seeing that food, water and shelter are sufficient to continue biological existence) only have a point when such an existence now or perhaps in the future again seems desirable.

Inevitably, our experiences are biosocial. It is the social setting which gives us the opportunity for most of the experiences we may or may not want to have. Having a life is the necessary condition for availing oneself of any opportunities which the social setting may offer. But having equitable access to a 'fair share of the opportunity range' (Daniels, 1985) which our particular society has to offer and of which reasonable persons may want to avail themselves, requires far more than merely having a life. If persons are to have a life as reasonably full as their biology permits, other things are needed.

This is analogous to the relationship between social justice and individual rights: individual rights without social justice are possible only for those fortunate enough to have their first order needs assured; those less lucky (those whose first order needs remain unmet and who, for example, are homeless or starving) will find their individual rights to be a cynical mockery. On the other hand, social justice alone is insufficient: life without individual rights becomes almost pointless. Social justice forms the necessary condition for a full life but without decent individual rights social justice alone is empty. Social justice, in that sense, is the necessary condition for the meaningful existence of individual rights.

In modern, industrialized societies access to a full opportunity range necessarily depends upon having reasonable health (and, if one happens not to have reasonable health, upon having access to reasonable health services) as well as upon sufficient education. Without at least some education persons not only cannot hope to aspire to a fulfilling life, they cannot even hope to recognize what a fulfilling life might be. Without an opportunity to sufficient education, a full range of opportunity which a person's talents and interests would otherwise enable them to have remains closed. Likewise, in modern societies health care is necessary if persons are to enjoy equal access commensurate with their talents and interests. Health care, including preventive medical care, is very much a part of modern society: dying or being seriously affected by a preventable, treatable or curable disease certainly constricts the reasonable opportunity range. Some may not require health care; many, however, will need a greater or lesser amount. The person whose vision without glasses is poor or who cannot walk without crutches; the diabetic; the person who develops pneumonia—all are obvious examples. Access to the full opportunity range in a modern, industrialized society is unthinkable without access to health care.

Beyond this, the concepts of health, disease, illness and death are things deeply buried in the very marrow of human existence. Therefore, these concepts are intimately and directly involved with very elemental human concerns: with suffering, birth, death, grief and joy. In our modern society, health care can significantly affect all of these. Health care is a quite different commodity than are TV sets, theatre tickets or washing machines. These neither seriously affect the opportunity range nor deal with things deeply buried in the very marrow of human existence.

Health care, in addition, is often care for conditions directly or indirectly produced by the way society has structured itself. Some advance the claim that illness and health are merely part of the 'natural lottery', the 'luck of the draw' and a matter of pure chance (Engelhardt, 1981). Others hold that, especially when it comes to sickness and health, the natural lottery is a social construct (Loewy, 1988a). Causality, especially in today's world, is a complex thing. Not only are mining coal, driving cars and working in chemical factories a function of the way in which communities have seen fit to structure themselves, illnesses other than those directly job-related likewise are inextricably intertwined with factors under communal control. Over and over again it has been shown that illness and health bear an important relationship to poverty, education and other social factors (Kosa and Zola, 1975; Fuchs, 1983; US Department of Commerce, 1980; Physician's Task Force on Hunger in America, 1985). In that respect too, health care is not a commodity quite like all other commodities.

Some see health care as a commodity like any other commodity, rightly purchasable by those fortunate enough to have the means to do so and not purchasable by those who do not (Engelhardt, 1988). Not having the means may be unfortunate but it is no one else's fault except perhaps the fault of the person who lacks the means (Engelhardt, 1981). Some societies, furthermore, seem not to attach as great a value to health care as do others: Engelhardt's (1986) Ba Mbuti are an example. In the state of nature in which the Ba Mbuti live, first order necessities remain the same but second order necessities may be quite different. For primitive people the full opportunity range which reasonable members of their society would want to attain is obviously not the same as it might be in industrialized nations. Since the full opportunity range for reasonable members of primitive societies differs markedly from the range in the industrialized world, the second order necessities of more primitive people, socially conditioned as are all second order necessities, are, therefore, also not the same. The fact that the Ba Mbuti (or members of some other starkly different constituted society) have no particular regard for health care is interesting, but it is uniquely uninformative when it comes to looking at our own problems.

If one believes that the natural lottery or chance alone chooses who will and who will not be ill or healthy, one may feel that communities, in justice, owe health care to all, or one may feel that since communities have no causal role in sickness and health no such obligation exists. Which of these points of view is adopted depends largely upon the way we look upon the structure of community.

4. LOOKING AT COMMUNITY

Even if we grant that health care is special, a commodity like few others, why should we, therefore, be inclined to see to it that all members of the community have, at the very least, a decent minimum? Are we, to the best of our ability, obliged to try and supply basic necessities to all? Our answer to these questions is largely determined by the way in which we view our social contract, community and justice.

The notion of social contract is an old one. Social contract consists of the tacit agreements which unite social structures (be they families, tribes or states) into functioning and cohesive wholes. Social contract consists of those things which 'go without saying' and which we consider to be the legitimate expectations we have of others and of our community. It underpins laws and cements communities. Without tacit social contract there can be no other understandings.

Notions of social contract can be found in Plato, in the Stoa and throughout medieval philosophy. In modern times social contract was first explicated by Hobbes (1962) who saw individuals as emerging from behind their rock to make a covenant motivated merely by terror. Individuals, prior to this, lived in a pre-social state of nature constantly in fear of each other and for their lives. At best, life was 'solitary, nasty, brutish and short'. Such pre-social people afraid for their own individual lives formed a covenant based on terror and founded solely on an agreement to refrain from doing each other physical harm. The stability of such a covenant promising mutual non-harm was assured by absolute obedience to a sovereign. A Hobbesian view of social contract leads to a minimalist concept of community: community consists of individuals pledged not to harm each other but in no way obligated to come to each other's aid. This idea is what underpins Nozick's (1974) vision of a minimalist community—a community in which freedom and autonomy are conditions instead of values of the moral life.

Locke (1980) saw social contract differently: social contract was a contract of evolving trust uniting equally free men. It was justified by an appeal to 'natural law' ultimately resting on 'God's will'. Keeping such a covenant implied more than merely mutual non-harm and it did not require an omnipotent sovereign. Rousseau (1968) takes this one step further: in his view, social structures create individual morality. Individuals can only be properly appreciated within the nexus of their social connections. As with Locke, such associations do far more than merely prevent harm: they actively promote 'good', which Rousseau sees as a social 'good' incomprehensible outside the social nexus. Still, even in Rousseau's view, it is individuals who initially covenant and, therefore, individuals remain ontologically prior to community.

One can look at social contract in other ways. Instead of seeing individuals as covenanting with one another only after emerging from a pre-political state of nature, a pre-social state as a necessary condition of such a contract may not be acknowledged (Loewy, 1988a, 1989). Men can be seen as always having huddled together, be it in families or in looser and more tribal associations. Far from being initially motivated by terror, agreements can be seen as having been motivated by mutual needs, trust and, inescapably, by biosocial interdependence. The very notion of non-harm to one another must be seen as underwritten by trust if it is to come about in the first place or if it is to endure in the final analysis (Loewy, 1988a). Unless there is at least minimal trust, men would not budge from behind their rock; unless there is mutual need (of which the need for protection from possible harm by others in the group is only a small part), no impulse to enter an association exists (Loewy, 1988a). A far greater than merely minimalist viewpoint of community emerges from such a concept. When needs, trust and biosocial interdependence, rather than merely terror, underwrite the contract, men are obligated to have at least some regard for the welfare of others.

When one looks at social contract in a non-Hobbesian way, the question of whether communities or individuals enjoy ontological priority becomes a 'chicken and egg' question: the one cannot be imagined without the other. Individuals are born into and reared by communities, suffused with communal values and shaped by communal customs. As, however, individual life experiences bring about changes in the individual, individuals in turn shape communities. The evolution of the individual is as incomprehensible outside the community as the community is incomprehensible without the individual.

If we accept a Hobbesian view of social contract, a minimalist community emerges. In such a community (as envisaged by Nozick) freedom and autonomy are absolutes. They are conditions and not values of the moral life (Engelhardt, 1986; Pellegrino and Thomasma, 1988). When autonomy is an absolute it can be restricted only when and if its free exercise threatens the free exercise of autonomy by another. Although some in such a community may consider beneficence to be nice, it has no moral standing and is an entirely supererogatory obligation. We and our communities are obliged not to prevent individuals from defining and meeting their own individual needs; but we and our communities are neither entitled to define what such needs are nor obligated to meet any of them. Persons are free to do exactly what they choose as long as doing so does not abrogate the same right for others. No motivational foundations or obligations of beneficence emerge from an autonomy-based ethic.

If we accept a more generous definition of community and accept obligations of beneficence as well as obligations of mutual non-harm, a different kind of world emerges. As Pellegrino and Thomasma (1988) have so forcefully pointed out, a decent regard for autonomy necessarily emerges from beneficence: one cannot be truly beneficent without a proper regard for the wishes and values of others. But the regard for autonomy is far from absolute. Autonomy and individual rights on the one hand are in tension with communal obligations on the other hand. From this dialectic, a synthesis defining the particular ethos of a particular community at a particular time emerges. The pendulum may swing either way but communities conceived in this way can evolve and grow whereas communities with an absolute regard for autonomy remain inflexible and fixed. When communities which hold freedom to be an absolute finally find that change is necessary for self-preservation (and when, therefore, they find it necessary to toss their inflexible principles overboard) they are more likely to abandon any regard for autonomy.

In a well accepted Aristotelian dictum, justice consists of giving everyone their due. What is and what is not someone's due, however, is another matter. Minimalist communities which see themselves as underwritten by a social contract forged in terror and which consequently accept freedom as an absolute condition of the moral life will see what is due quite differently than will more generously based communities. What is due in minimalist communities is doing each other no harm; what is due in broader-based communities is a far more difficult matter and one which will ultimately be determined by an ongoing dialectic between communal values and individual interests.

5. OBLIGATIONS IN MODERN COMMUNITIES

If we accept an entirely autonomy-based ethic, little else need be said. Such communities have no beneficent obligations towards their members and consequently can have no other obligations when it comes to first or second order needs, except to see to it that no one directly interferes with another's access. They have no right to tax the wealthy (unless the wealthy individually, for whatever reason, consent to be taxed!) and no obligation or funds to provide first or second order needs to their members.

The basic idea of the libertarian or Nozickian position is flawed in principle as well as consequence, for a number of reasons. First of all, the way Hobbes and some others envision a pre-social condition defies both evidence and reason. Hobbes' notion of contract based merely on terror and devoid of trust is flawed firstly, because individuals were never solitary and secondly, because terror of one another could not have been the sole (or, perhaps, even the most important) motivating force.

Persons, as I have already said, were never solitary: necessarily, individual existence started in family groups and from family groups kinship groups inevitably and probably simultaneously emerged. Solitary man roaming the earth looking out for himself and in absolute terror of his fellows doesn't quite ring true. At the very least, humans lived in families, were nurtured, protected and reared in the embrace of others and, inevitably, were suffused with the particular values of their group. And undoubtedly small kinship groups lived together—all evidence points that way. To live together, whether in families, kinship groups, tribes or large associations, requires complex implicit mutual understandings beyond a simple compact of mutual non-harm.

The genesis of our initial contract cannot, as Hobbes would have it, originate solely in terror. So that covenanting could take place, an implicit understanding concerning the possibility of covenant and notions of covenant keeping had to be about. One person may have feared another, as may one family or kinship group and that may have helped to motivate a compact in which mutual non-harm was an important feature. To reach such a compact, however; to come out, as it were, from behind the rock or tree to covenant, at least minimal trust must be presumed. Mutually agreeing not to harm each other when we do not expect others to feel any urgency to keep the compact does not make much sense. Furthermore, families and kinship groups had needs quite apart from the need to be left alone to pursue their own individualistic ends: they had needs for mutual protection not from each other but from the forces of nature about them. Such needs were more readily met when individuals stood together to help (not merely in order not to harm) each other. There is ample evidence that individual ends in early associations were inevitably subjugated to communal needs. The insistence on individual autonomy is, historically, a rather modern preoccupation.

Hobbes' contract is conceptually interesting. It necessarily underpins a libertarian notion of absolute respect for persons, strict individualism and, perhaps, underlines the need for an absolute sovereign if stark individualism is to play itself out. In that sense, absolutism and autocracy can be seen to be carried by the Trojan horse of freedom (Loewy, 1987b). If one accepts a Hobbesian notion of initial contract, a minimalist ethic in which freedom and autonomy are conditions and not values of the moral life ('side constraints' as Nozick would have it) necessarily emerges. Our initial contract is based four-square on the guarantee of mutual non-harm and on nothing else. We are obligated to our fellows in so far as we are not allowed to injure them and, by inference, in so far as mutual, freely entered contract specifies—but by nothing else. Ideas of beneficence to each other, notions of mutual help, communal obligations, all are without moral force. Private individuals or idiosyncratic moral enclaves may freely assume such obligations for themselves but they have no wider standing and cannot, in the larger community, be enforced. Such communities, I will argue, are not only flawed in their conception: they are also defective because they are inflexible, practically self-destroying and simply not what we think of when we say 'community'.

Communities with a monolithic devotion to individual freedom do not have the capacity to trade values in the market place of values. There is no dialectic between individual obligation and communal needs; no ability to change with time and circumstance when it comes to taking from one and giving to the other value; no capacity to learn by past error and to grow into future betterment. Inquiry into the moral life ceases to be a 'making of the indeterminate a little more determinate' (Dewey, 1938). Rather, it is a monolithic pursuit of one end: personal freedom restricted only by the need not directly to injure others. Respecting persons by allowing them (involuntarily) to starve to death or by failing to facilitate their access to the good things society may offer is a strange and cold sort of respect. And facilitating others in such communities is not a moral obligation; only not directly causing harm is.

The inflexibility that results leads to the untrammelled accumulation of material goods by some to the detriment of others and, inevitably, will lead to the domination of the weak by the strong, the poor by the wealthy (Niebuhr, 1957). A society shaped in this way has an ever-present danger, indeed a certainty, of ever-growing class war until violence is made almost inevitable. The poor are not apt to starve forever for the sake of an abstract idea, especially of an abstract idea already flawed in its inception. Societies in which there can be an ongoing dialectic between the needs of individuals and the needs of the community can make compromises and place a different emphasis on different values at different times; societies that lack flexibility are prone to break instead of bending (Loewy, 1988b).

Inflexible societies are self-destructive. They cannot adapt, change or learn from experience when it comes to adopting a new course. In minimalist societies individual liberty can be infringed only with the personal consent of those infringed: those, for example, unwilling to be taxed can opt out. To say the least, the practicality of such a course of action is questionable. Few of us love to pay taxes or engage in community work, even when we might be willing to do so provided our neighbour necessarily suffers under the same handicap. Even in prehistoric times, associations had communal biosocially determined needs which only communal action could accomplish; in the modern world, larger communities of inevitably closely connected people have even greater common needs which only communal action can hope to fulfil. Whether we like it or not, our larger communities are taking on a global complexion: at least some mutual world-needs (especially when it comes to things such as food production, communication, safety or public health) exist today and more will exist tomorrow. We need to recognize that our mutual terror (our fear of dying in a nuclear holocaust, for example) does not suffice to ensure stability. A minimalist community, one in which my neighbour and I are both free to produce and own (but perhaps not use!) any weapon or system we care to, simply cannot even prevent the mutual terror it was intended to prevent. Such a philosophy can easily introduce world destruction.

Lastly, community in ordinary language is a complex notion. When we speak of it, in any language, more than merely non-harm comes to mind. It is a notion which is far more than merely negative and includes concepts of nurture and benefit. Beneficence and trust must underpin all lasting associations even though beneficence may, at times, not be evident and trust may, at other times, be violated. Nevertheless, the very fact of decrying an absence of beneficence and recognizing a breach of trust speaks for the prior existence of such virtues. From trust and beneficence, respect for autonomy must necessarily emerge: one cannot be truly beneficent, or truly care for the good of other persons without caring and respecting the values held by them (Pellegrino and Thomasma, 1988). Autonomy and respect for persons is a necessary condition of acting beneficently; autonomy, on the other hand, does not entail any regard for the good of others. When we speak of community we almost invariably have more in mind than an uncaring monolithic regard for another's autonomy; inevitably we see in the notion of community the necessity of advancing the good of others as well as our own. Solidarity and community are much more broadly conceived than is suggested by an autonomy-based, monolithic, minimalist ethic.

I will assume that communities cannot (and in fact do not) adopt a completely minimalist viewpoint. If communities are conceded to be more than minimalist, what remains is to show exactly what, beyond the minimal obligation of non-interference, communities owe to their members and what individual members owe to each other. If communities are to be even minimally beneficent, first order necessities for all would be the first order of business. The most minimal beneficence would try to sustain life: less than that would no longer be beneficent. If communities have beneficent obligations towards their members (and if the members have beneficent obligations towards each other) these obligations must be founded on a bedrock of providing first order needs. Unless such bare necessities of life are assured, assuring anything beyond makes no sense. Funds for supplying such bare necessities are, of course, ultimately derived by taxing those who can best afford to contribute. Doing this inevitably interferes with the freedom of some so that the existence of others can be assured. Allowing some members of the community the enjoyment of opulence while others starve or freeze violates the definition of justice implied by anything beyond a minimalist community. If justice is to give to each what is his or her due and if the idea of what is due flows from the viewpoint of community we choose to adopt, then a community which sees itself as obligated beyond merely refraining from harm will adopt measures designed to implement at least minimal beneficence. If it fails to do so, its claim to being at least minimally beneficent vanishes.

I have argued that second order necessities are socially defined. Further, I have argued that there are basic second order necessities which are basic because fulfilling them enables one to have access to a full opportunity range. It is the meeting of second order necessities which makes meeting first order necessities worthwhile. Without having access to at least a decent share of some of the good things in life is hardly meaningful. When basic second order needs are not met, persons often not only cannot attain a fair opportunity range but lose all hope of doing so. In many ways, social justice is the necessary condition for individual rights analogous to the way that life is the necessary condition for experience. Beneficence, in that sense, is the necessary condition for meaningful autonomy.

Minimally beneficent communities may argue that once they have assured a minimal physical existence to all (once they have, in other words, met first order needs) no further obligation to provide access to the good things in life exists. Communities which argue this way condemn themselves to an almost fixed class system in which only a few exceptionally talented and exceptionally lucky persons can ever emerge from those born into ignorance, poverty and disease. They begin to live in a state in which the opportunity range of their class is not even seen to overlap with the opportunity range of others. In effect, such persons cannot even imagine themselves as gaining positions to which others easily aspire. Assuring those born into such a state merely of an opportunity to exist and of nothing more creates a system in which a large and inevitably growing segment of the population is in hopeless despair. Such persons, history has shown, can be held down only by force and then only for a finite length of time. Meeting basic second order needs (in our kind of society at least full educational opportunity and health care) can help to prevent such a state of affairs. Basic second order needs are not commodities like TV sets, theatre tickets or washing machines and, therefore, market distribution and entrepreneurial profit-taking for meeting such needs is quite a different matter. Taxing those who can best afford to pay, even if this decreases their ability to live in extreme luxury and opulence, in order to assure that the basic second order necessities of all will be met, seems commensurate with a definition of justice emerging from a view of community believing not only in minimal but in somewhat more than minimal beneficence.

In our own time, there has inevitably been a communal dialectic between individual rights and communal obligations. No nation has ever completely succeeded in eliminating all individual rights or in having its citizens live an entirely individualistic existence. The Soviet Union, emphasizing communal obligations, paid woefully little attention to individuals and to their rights (except, perhaps, when these individuals were members of the bureaucracy); the United States, priding itself on the possibilities for the individual which its system offered, paid scant attention to social justice issues (except when those who were well-off one day found themselves out on the street the next). One system led to the community of the Gulag; the other to the individual freedom to starve to death in the street.

The dialectic between communal interests and individual rights in the United States has, for a variety of reasons, strongly favoured individual rights. The result has been a state of affairs in which homelessness, hunger, lack of health care, inferior primary and shrinking access to higher education have become the order of the day. If the nation is wise, the dialectic may swing the other way: even within the medical community there is an ever-growing acceptance that some form of social medicine is inevitable and indeed desirable. Unfortunately, wisdom does not seem to be the order of the day: powerful forces are opposed to a more communitarian approach and these forces currently seem to control the mechanisms of government.

The United States as well as other communities will have to make its own choice. Communities wishing to pursue a crass capitalist philosophy, perhaps slightly ameliorated by assuring that minimal basic first order needs are met, will find themselves discomfited by an ever-growing underclass of the disadvantaged. Such communities court their own destruction: inevitably as the numbers of the unfortunate grow, their pressure upon the rest of society increases until, and again inevitably, it erupts. The hordes of the ill fed, ill housed and ill clad (not to speak of those poorly educated and in marginal or poor health) are not apt to make wise and well reasoned choices. To speak of 'democracy' in such communities is cynical. On the other hand, more generous communities which see their obligation as at least providing fair access to the good things of life and which, therefore, are inclined to meet the basic second order needs of their members as part of their particular social contract, can grow and thrive. A few individual members in such communities may, perhaps, not be able to enjoy quite as opulent or luxurious a lifestyle; but all will have a fair chance to lead an enjoyable and fulfilling life. Since such communities will deal with a far happier and more willing constituency, change can be accomplished more smoothly and more peacefully. Communities of this sort can grow and enjoy a true democracy in which a well informed, basically healthy and caring membership can determine its own destiny.

REFERENCES

Churchill, L. R. (1987) *Rationing Health-Care in America: Perceptions and Principles of Justice*. University of Notre Dame Press, Notre Dame.

Daniels, N. (1985) *Just Health Care*. Cambridge University Press, New York.

Dewey, J. (1938) *Logic, the Theory of Inquiry*. Henry Holt, New York.

Engelhardt, H. T. (1981) Health care allocations: responses to the unjust, the unfortunate and the undesireable. In: Shelp, E. E. (ed.). *Justice and Health Care*. D. Reidel, Dordrecht, Holland.

Engelhardt, H. T. (1986) *The Foundations of Bioethics*. Oxford University Press, New York.

Engelhardt, H. T. (1988) Morality for the medical–industrial complex: a code of ethics for the mass-marketing of health-care. *New England Journal of Medicine* **319**, 1086–9.

Fuchs, V. R. (1983) *Economic Aspects of Health*. University of Chicago Press, Chicago, IL.
Hobbes, T. (1962) *Leviathan*. Collier Books, New York.
Kosa, J., Zola, I. K. (1975) *Poverty and Health: A Sociological Analysis*. Harvard University Press, Cambridge, MA.
Locke, J. (1980) *Second Treatise of Government*. Hackett Publishing, Indianapolis, IN.
Loewy, E. H. (1987a) Treatment decisions in the mentally impaired: limiting but not abandoning treatment. *New England Journal of Medicine* **317**, 1465–69.
Loewy, E. H. (1987b) Not by reason alone: a review of H. Tristram Engelhardt's *Foundations of Bioethics*. *Journal of Medicine, Humanities and Bioethics* **8**, 67–72.
Loewy, E. H. (1988a) Communities, self-causation and the natural lottery. *Social Sciences and Medicine* **26**, 1133–9.
Loewy, E. H. (1988b) AIDS and the human community. *Social Sciences and Medicine* **27**, 297–303.
Loewy, E. H. (1989) *A Textbook of Medicine Ethics*. Plenum Publishers, New York.
Niebuhr, R. (1957) Rationing and democracy. In: *Love and Justice*. (Robertson, D. R. ed.). Westminster Press, Philadelphia, PA.
Nozick, R. (1974) *Anarchy, State and Utopia*. Basic Books, New York.
Pellegrino, E. D. and Thomasma, D. C. (1988) *For the Patient's Good: The Restoration of Beneficence in Health Care*. Oxford University Press, New York.
Physician's Task Force on Hunger in America (1985) *Hunger in America*. Wesleyan University Press, Middletown, CT.
Rachels, J. (1986) *The End of Life*. Oxford University Press, New York.
Rousseau, J. J. (1968) *The Social Contract*. (Transl: Cranston, M.) Penguin Books, Baltimore, MD.
US Department of Commerce (1980) *Social Indicators*. Government Printing Office, Washington, DC.

3

Changing Conceptions of Medical Ethics

Henk ten Have and Gerrit Kimsma

Medical ethics nowadays seems to be in a state of paradox. Moral issues tend to multiply more rapidly every day, but professional ethicists are relatively unsuccessful in resolving these issues. The media are taking a tremendous interest in the moral problems of health care, but the effect of ethical debate on decisions in clinical medicine, nursing care and public policy is limited.

Medical technology is usually regarded as one of the major sources of moral problems in modern medicine, but the overwhelming majority of ethical studies concentrate more on the conditions for application of new technologies than on the conditions for their creation and development. In short, these observations illustrate the substantial discrepancy between the public attention paid to moral questions and the actual impact of ethics on the common practices of medicine as well as the direction of the development of medicine.

1. AUTONOMOUS TECHNOLOGY

Since the middle of the 19th century, science and technology in general have been central to the changing face of western medicine. Medicine has changed through technology, either as a result of the impact of non-medical technology on society, through improvement in hygiene, food and housing, or through the impact of medical technologies per se, making possible what formerly existed only in dreams and fantasy. As a result of the first effect, a change in disease patterns emerged from the treatable acute and infectious diseases to chronic diseases whose effects can be ameliorated only marginally.

Changing Values in Medical and Health Care Decision Making
Edited by U. J. Jensen and G. Mooney

The second phenomenon, medical technology itself, has added greatly to the realisation that, in the words of David Greaves (1979), the medical enterprise is in need of reappraisal. Not only is medical technology blamed for its impersonal and inhumane nature, but increasingly the goals, direction and effectiveness of technological medicine have come to be questioned. In addition to these undeniably serious matters, the social role of medical professionals and the areas in society that should be dealt with by medicine—the subject of medicalisation of society—are increasingly under scrutiny. And to make this description complete, the change in social attitudes, towards technology in general and medicine specifically, results in a change in attitudes towards medical professionals in particular and an increasing demand on the part of society to partake in medical decision making at all levels, ranging from the individual doctor–patient encounter to the structure of the health care system. This demand more and more starts with the basic tenet that the medical enterprise is too badly administered and costs increase beyond control.

Within the analysis of these problems encircling medicine, the thesis of the autonomy of technology plays an important part. And it must be said that it is tempting to blame the autonomy of technology for the frustrating problems in health care and the related inability and weaknesses of ethical discourse in medicine to do anything about it. Apparently the belief that technology has gone out of control and is following its own course, independent of human direction or management, is attractive. This thesis of the 'technological temptation' seems effectively to rule out other alternatives and actions. This for example becomes clear in the analysis of the French philosopher Jacques Ellul in his study on the technological society (Ellul, 1954), which describes six characteristics of modern technique that seem to apply almost uniformly to medical technology.

1. The first one is an *automatism of technical choice,* implying that human beings no longer perceive themselves as agents of choice in the means to be employed. For medicine this translates to an overwhelming choice for technical strategies of care instead of personal ones.
2. The aspect of *self-augmentation,* meaning that in a given civilisation technical progress is irreversible. Technology tends to act not according to arithmetic but to geometric progression, forcing technical changes in related areas of social activity.
3. The technical phenomenon leads to *monism* in form and approach, resulting in a blotting out of differences, whether they be personal or institutional, moral or religious.
4. The *necessary linking together of techniques,* meaning a necessary expansion and 'radiation' of technological conditions and procedures throughout society as a whole, is the result of the implementation of single inventions.

5. Technology leads to *technical universalism*, both geographically and qualitatively.
6. *Technique develops in an autonomous fashion* where, for the technique, external conditions no longer determine its development and direction.

Similar ideas have been expressed by other modern philosophers. According to Martin Heidegger (1966), for example, in his *Discourse on Thinking* man's own technical creations have outgrown his capacity for decision. He points out that 'technological advance will move faster and faster and can never be stopped', echoing in a way the Faustian theme of the spirit let out of the bottle, turning against the human quality of civilisation.

Medicine even has had its own anti-technology paradigm in the appearance of Illich's *Medical Nemesis* (1975). Its dominant theme is the impersonality of technical care and the devious destruction by the medical profession, through technology, of the individuals' ability for cure and care, creating an addiction to medical technological solutions.

These ideas, however valuable they may be analytically, have a limited effect on our ability to redirect these developments or to make a change for the better. Even though it is granted first that the conventional view of a neutrality of technology—no more than tools or means to desired ends—is not tenable, and second that technology is advancing certain ends while denying others, leading to a revaluation of values during this process of technicalisation of western culture, ethical approaches show an apparent lack of power to control technology in general, medical technology included.

The loss of mastery of technology manifests itself in a corresponding loss of moral command. This is a process that can be closely observed in the developments in modern health care. The medical technologies that have extended man's control over disease, life, and the human body are themselves dictating their norms and requirements. They generate technicised definitions of human ends and substitute technical solutions for problems that were moral in nature.

This notion of autonomous technology would seem to make a great deal of sense. It is consistent with many experiences in modern life. But far from being controlled by the desired and rational ends of human beings, technology now appears to govern its own course. However, this is true only to a certain extent, unless we are prepared to embrace the doctrine of technological determinism.

Some aspects of the process of technical change do depend on the elements of free will and conscious decision. Even though not everything is possible and some limits have been set, it does not follow that it is pointless to make decisions and choices. The problem is, as the critics have argued, that our capacity to make free choices to control technological development has itself been eroded by an attachment to the mode of technological change, and that technologies give structure to our conception of human needs and ends themselves. Each of us lives with procedures, roles, institutions that are not of our own making but that nevertheless powerfully shape what we do. Many of our decisions reflect adaptive responses instead of real choices.

2. ETHICS

What has this to do with the current situation of medical ethics? Much more than is evident at first sight. It is our conviction and conclusion that ethics is not and should not be conceived as being subordinated to the relative autonomy of technology, but rather that it has lost its moral command because it has itself become part and parcel of the technological order. And even this evaluation is not immediately clear to the observer, because medical ethics seems in a state of paradox. On the one hand, there is an accumulated necessity, an increased attention and high visibility for ethics. On the other hand however, this increased attention is relatively ineffective and ethical proposals carry little weight in day-to-day and policy decisions. Ethics has become powerless, probably because it is itself governed by the idea of technical rationality (the accommodation of means to ends). It has been transformed into a techno-ethics, a kind of *technethics*.

Our thesis is that in the last two decades a conception and practice of ethics has emerged that understands itself as a separate discipline disconnected from philosophy as well as medicine. And this concept and practice, as a discipline, has paradoxically become vested with the same ideological functions as the traditional professional codes. Since it is primarily concerned with legitimising and facilitating medical progress we could not expect present-day ethics to criticise the values of medicine and health care or to scrutinise with anticipation the desirability and utility of medical and technological innovations. The problem is that this prevailing conception of ethics is itself impregnated with the idea of technical rationality; and the question is whether a different conception of ethics can be developed that is less dependent on this technological imperative.

We will try to show that such an alternative approach is possible by comparing two conceptions of medical ethics as they are currently in use or in vogue—the new approach of so-called clinical ethics and the current approach of applied ethics.

3. APPLIED ETHICS

Since the late sixties medical ethics has been redefined as *applied ethics*. This self-image of ethics is obvious and foundational for the mainstream of professional literature. In Beauchamp and Childress's *Principles of Biomedical Ethics* (1983), biomedical ethics is defined as 'the application of general ethical theories, principles and rules to problems of therapeutic practice, health care delivery, and medical and biological research'.

This definition illustrates why medical ethics is perceived as a specific discipline: there is a set of moral principles and ethical theories that should apply to a variety of biomedical problems. The context in which these problems arise is not peculiar in the sense of being characterised by intrinsic values which generate special problems. On the contrary, the medical context is seen as a sort of practice ground for a new profession of self-styled ethicists. The expertise claimed by them is threefold:

1. *Mastery of ethical theory*. Ethicists claim to possess a body of knowledge concerning ethical traditions and theories that can be utilised to solve moral problems arising in medical practice.
2. *Conceptual clarification*, i.e. the skill of analysing the meaning of concepts, of detecting fallacies and exposing invalid arguments. By this analytical dissection of the issues all components of medical decision making can be clarified and structured, in particular the ethical principles involved and the central concepts used.
3. *Impartiality in weighing alternatives*. The analysing and structuring just mentioned are supposed to produce a road map, if we are to believe the American ethicist Danner Clouser (1975). Ethics 'shows where various arguments and actions lead, what facts would be relevant, what concepts are crucial, and what moral principles are at issue, and probably in conflict'. This is the central contribution of medical ethics. It does not necessarily result in a judgment on what we should do. The ethicist gives us the topography of arguments, and objectifies the options. He regards himself as a disinterested and neutral observer of medical practice, who is in the best position to weigh alternatives.

3.1. Criticism

These three elements of moral expertise have brought into existence a type of medical ethics which is pertinently described by Arthur Caplan (1982) as 'the engineering model of applied ethics'.

In recent years this concept of medical ethics has been the cause of more and more discontent, primarily among practising physicians. They complain about a biomedical ethics establishment, led by non-physicians having an anti-medicine bias, who nevertheless produce ethical positions that are turned into legal and public policy changes affecting the practice of medicine. These sentiments are motivated by a concern to increase the involvement of physicians in medical ethics and to focus attention on the routine moral problems within the daily interactions of doctors and patients. Gradually, the theoretical basis for a new conception of medical ethics has been constructed. It is the result of a critical questioning of the presuppositions of the conception of applied ethics.

1. Can it be assumed that there is a body of knowledge about normative ethical theories that can be applied in medical settings? Or stated otherwise: is medical ethics just the application of principles to cases? This presupposition has firm roots both in old-time foundationalist ethics and philosophy of science: the belief that there is a rock bottom of first principles or a priori truths, or in the case of philosophy of science, a natural order of things, an objective reality apart from the observers or actors upon which the edifice of ethics and science can be erected.

   In the field of philosophy of science however this view has been challenged and abandoned, especially through research in quantum physics. Here the idea of an objective reality or natural order has become more and more remote since, amongst others, Heisenberg made clear that the idea of an objective reality must be replaced by the representation of our *knowledge of this reality*. In quantum physics, it appears that the smaller the particles we try to describe, the more the method of discovery interferes with their processes. This implies the necessity to include the observer in any theory of reality and a bankruptcy of a reality outside the observing eye. In this confrontation with reality, man is confronted more and more not with nature but with his own artificial structures and products. It means also that increasingly we have to realise the untenability of a separation of object from methodology, because our approaches change the objects.

   The same line of reasoning can be adopted for medical ethics. The idea that a body of knowledge of normative theories describes the reality of and in medicine implies a separation of ethical theory and medical practice, even a precedence of theory over practice. It implies further the absence of normative considerations in actual medical decision making. This however not only does not hold true for physics, as Heisenberg (1971) explained, but certainly cannot be defended for medical ethics. More than 100 years before Heisenberg, the existentialist philosopher Kierkegaard (1978) already contended the same when he observed that 'a change takes place in the knower when he has to apply his knowledge'. Ethics, after all, is not only a product (viz. a collection of prescriptions for professional conduct) but essentially a process (viz. a systematic and continuous reflection on the norms and values guiding medical theory and practice).

   From this point of view, moral concerns evolve within medical settings themselves and are a function of the roles involved, e.g. patients and physicians. From here two conclusions are clear:

a. the normative empiricism of medical practices must be taken into account, more than the conformity of these practices with pre-existing ethical theories;
b. morality is something we all participate in; medical ethics in particular is not the result of esoteric knowledge; anyone involved in the medical setting is a moral participant and expert in at least intuitive knowledge and notions.

2. The second presupposition that has been criticised is the belief that the application of moral knowledge is merely a process of deduction. Even this belief is a relic of an old model from philosophy of science: the model of *deductive–nomological explanation*. Moral data are explained by subsuming them under a set of moral principles, just as a scientific explanation may be conceived as a deductive argument whose explanatory statements consist of general laws and descriptions of particular facts, and whose conclusion follows from subsumption under those laws.

   But in medical practice moral issues are not self-evident. What is perceived and described as a moral datum is not independent of theoretical and practical preconceptions but dependent on what we perceive as goals and intentions. We need to know more about the processes and reasons of interpreting and defining problems in specific health care settings explicitly as *moral* problems.

4. CLINICAL ETHICS

These criticisms have given rise to a different practice of ethics, based on a new conception of medical ethics: *clinical ethics*. It is defined by Jonsen *et al*. (1986) as: 'the identification, analysis and resolution of moral problems that arise in the care of a particular patient'.

The extent to which clinical ethics differs from the current conception of applied ethics can be summarised under four headings:

1. *Insider perspective*: In formulating a clinical decision the physician must take into account the ethical dimension. As a result of the special nature of the doctor–patient relationship he or she is not a mere observer but an involved participant. This means that the realities of clinical decision making are crucial for an understanding of the moral dimensions. The clinical ethical problems arising in the practice of surgery are not the same as those in paediatrics, or obstetrics and gynaecology. They are not of the same nature 'medically' but differ also with respect to the extent of risks and benefits. Specifically the insider's perspective allows for the estimation of whether risks are low in routine investigation or substantial

with questionable benefit. Clinicians are in the best position to identify moral issues in the context of the clinical situation. An 'insider' perspective is needed to direct attention to the routine ethical questions in clinical encounters, but even more to develop empirical data relating to the process and outcome of clinical encounters: How do patients and doctors actually make decisions? What moral options are involved? What are the effects of values in reaching decisions?

2. *Method of induction:* In contrast to an *ethica ordine geometrico demonstrata,* an ethics as a deductive process by which fundamental theories and principles are applied to practical moral dilemmas, an inductive methodology is being developed which starts with careful analysis of the empirical conditions. In this respect there is at the moment a renewed interest in classical casuistry (Jonsen and Toulmin, 1988). In the casuistical method there are paradigm cases in which a moral maxim is clearly applicable. Analogies are then constructed: cases in which, due to different circumstances, a moral maxim appears less suitable. There is thus a range from highly to less plausible arguments. The factual circumstances of a case are very relevant: they make different cases. The casuist's task is to determine the degree to which the relevant moral maxims fit the particular circumstances, but even more, which factors, personal preferences or environmental conditions are relevant enough to be judged as moral facts.

   In most cases the fit is not perfect; that means that the case is more or less convincing, probable or arguable, but not certain. The casuistic approach corresponds largely to the analogical reasoning used in clinical decision making. In diagnosis, therapy and prognosis the clinician matches by analogy the case of a patient with other cases presented in textbooks, classical descriptions or pathological theories. Like clinicians, the casuist aims not only at understanding a moral problem but at resolving it; he or she offers advice about the action which seems to be most appropriate in these particular circumstances. Unlike other ethicists, however, he or she organises his or her ethical approach, not around philosophical or moral principles, but around clusters of factual circumstances relevant to medical decisions such as patient preferences or medical indications.

3. *Interdependence of technical and normative dimensions of clinical judgment*: This interdependence, which is at the basis of clinical ethics, is repeatedly underlined by recent work in philosophy of medicine. It is argued that medicine is intrinsically a moral activity since it has a unique character as a healing relationship between doctor and patient. Value judgments are pervasive in clinical decisions. The moral concerns are therefore inseparable from the technical concerns about the correct diagnosis and the best treatment. Good medicine is necessarily ethical medicine. The New

York internist Eric Cassell (1976) has reaffirmed this old professional conviction, writing that medicine is inherently a moral profession whose tools are, in part, technical; he concludes: 'problems that do fall within the system of medicine are *also* moral matters because medical decisions affect not only the body but also the life and welfare of the patient'. Thus a moral–technical duality is fictitious: clinical decisions are ethical decisions.

4. *Ethics as an inherent reflective function of medicine itself:* This is the logical consequence of the ideas just mentioned. When physicians consider ethics as an intrinsic feature of their craft, then ethical analysis of medical decisions cannot proceed from an externally imposed system but is an inherent, second-order function of medicine. If a normative dimension is intrinsic to medical practice itself, physicians have an obligation to reflect on the moral quandaries of medicine.

   That implies among other things that the teaching of ethics to medical students can best be done by physicians. But then they will have to be prepared to transfer the traditional commitments of their art and science to future colleagues. It is of course true that this transfer of commitments in fact takes place in the clinic every day but thus far this transfer has been implicit and is not systematically reflected upon. Clinical ethics as a new approach will only succeed if there is an explicit teaching of medical ethics in the clinical setting by doctors themselves. The view must become common sense that most clinical decisions are not sound as long as the normative dimension is not explicated and discussed.

4.1. Examples

Let us give two examples to clarify our opposition. The first example is derived from the field of medical research, especially critical care medicine, and concerns the idea of autonomy. The second concerns tensions within the basic notion of informed consent, especially within primary care settings. Given the relatedness of the ideas of autonomy and informed consent, the examples are not exhaustive but illustrations of the practical impossibility of applied ethics as this becomes clear in research and common medical interventions.

Example 1

For medical research, according to the Declaration of Helsinki (1964) and subsequent revisions, the notion of patient approval after information is essential. This approval is based on the presupposition of competence, a competence that is rooted in the idea of the autonomy of the potential research subjects. On that basis, where there exists a limitation of autonomy or a diminution of competence in the face of an emergency situation, where the dependence on care is urgent, according to a strict interpretation of the Helsinki rules, no research would be possible. This would be true not only in cases of unconscious or comatose patients, but also in any emergency situation where the acute necessity of medical interventions makes it unacceptable to spend the time necessary to inform the patient. It would also hold when, in a situation of illness and pain, in the face of a diminished capacity to understand, even when there is no legal incompetence, the matter of liberty to decide on the basis of adequate information becomes fictitious. To reiterate: we are not talking about treatment decisions in emergency cases where the requirement for informed consent can legitimately be foregone, but about medical research.

This theoretical tension however does not impede critical care research. Even though theoretically it is not 'possible', in the face of potential benefits, it remains 'acceptable'. In the ethics literature, for example in Dworkin's *The Theory and Practice of Autonomy* (1988), this friction between principles and reality has been 'solved' by introducing the notions of 'weak' and 'strong' autonomy. These additional characterising qualifications may be a recognition of a medical reality. Conceptually they constitute a monstrosity without adequate guiding capacity, as they were meant to be. That means then both a continuation of necessary research for that category of patients and inadequate understanding and conceptualisation. Here the new conception of clinical ethics could give us better insight into what happens in practice. Especially the two notions of the insider's perspective, making particular evaluations possible of risks and benefits, and inductive, factual arguments that are relevant, play an important part and should theoretically be recognised. This recognition should have consequences for the description of the position and responsibility of the clinicians involved in research and lead to a further differentiation of types of research and ethical conditions.

Example 2

The second example concerns the adequacy of the principle of informed consent in medical practice. In a recent article, Howard Brody (1989) professes that 'the theory and the practice of informed consent are out of joint in some crucial ways'. The concept appears to be 'poorly integrated into American medical practice' and there is no reason to suppose that it has fared better in non-American medical settings. The reason for this imbalance between wish and reality, especially in primary care settings, is that the 'principled approach' of informed consent has been 'hardened' by the use of legal standards as an extension of ethical principles. The ethical principle implies informing a patient of the possible risks and potential benefits of medical interventions, whether these are diagnostic or therapeutic, in order to aid medical decision making. The legalistic interpretation of this duty by physicians implies that one must set out all possible risks as well as the benefits and alternatives. In practice this leads more to attention to completeness of information than to awareness about how this information was used in the process of decision making: 'To the physician obtaining informed consent, *you never know when you are finished*' (Brody, 1989). This conclusion may be valid especially for the American medical enterprise, with its heavy dependence on court interpretations. In principle it is the case that a fixed point cannot be established from which one can be certain that one has adequately completed one's legal as well as one's ethical task. In awareness of the shortcomings of this interpretation of informed consent, Jay Katz (1984) has proposed the introduction of a model of 'informed consent as conversation ', to reach a better integration of the principle into medical practice. The limitations of this model however are that the preponderance of subjective elements of a 'conversation' preclude an adequate retrospective check or review, especially in cases of conflict.

To overcome these shortcomings of both models, Brody proposes a new standard, the so-called 'transparency standard', that is the exact parallel of what we mean by the limitations of applied ethics and a renewal of clinical ethics. Transparency in this model means adequate disclosure to the patient of the physician's basic thinking and 'reconstructive' participation of the patient in asking questions and receiving answers, before the final decision has been made. This approach unquestionably integrates the exigencies of informed consent with the practice of medicine in general. It even allows for a differentiation between clinical and primary care settings, since it differentiates according to the seriousness of interventions. And it allows for retrospective evaluation of the adequacy of the process of information in case of legal intervention.

5. HERMENEUTIC ETHICS

5.1. The double face of clinical ethics

Along with the expansion of the teaching of medical ethics and with the rapidly increasing number of hospital ethics committees, clinical ethics has become very popular. But it is clear that for many ethicists 'clinical ethics' is not a notion denoting an alternative conception of medical ethics but rather a label specifying a particular field of application of ethical rules and principles. For them, clinical ethics simply means doing ethics in the clinical setting, without any necessity to change their conception and methods of applied ethics. Clinical ethics is then a special case of applied ethics. The initial impulse to re-orientate ethics is neutralised; the disadvantages of applied ethics can be overcome by introducing ethical discourse into the clinical world, and the same underlying values can be saved. Applied as well as clinical ethics can continue to emphasise values as technical rationality, regulation and universality. Doing so, they remain typical representatives of the Enlightenment and Modernity.

However, this strategy of assimilating clinical ethics into the standard notion of applied ethics misconstrues the post-modernist critique of western culture. The project of Modernity, in the view of Jean-François Lyotard (1986), is not unfinished or in need of expansion but it is bankrupt; its failures are intrinsic, not accidental but essential. The speculative discourses functioning as ideals of emancipation for mankind and used to legitimate scientific, philosophical and political practices are dead. As emancipation cannot legitimise present-day technoscience and technethics, their only legitimation nowadays is the enhancement of the 'performativity' (*performativité* in French) of the social system, i.e. its output and efficiency. Something is justifiable if it works; other criteria such as truth and justice are irrelevant. In post-modern society, the normative quality of laws and rules has been replaced by the functional quality of procedures. The system needs functionaries. It is therefore primarily interested in training competencies, and not any longer in Bildung, the shaping of characters or the propagating of ideals of life (Lyotard, 1986). The same characteristics can be observed in ethics: clinical ethicists as a new type of hospital functionary (requesting licensing and fee-for-service) and educational activities of hospital ethics committees aimed at training analytical and argumentative competencies in reviewing cases.

Such assimilation of clinical ethics to applied ethics ignores the criticisms referred to earlier in our discussion of applied ethics. Furthermore, on the basis of experience it is a well known fact that knowledge of philosophy and ethics is most of the time insufficient in the clinical setting. For example, utilitarianism could be interesting as a moral theory, but at the bedside a utilitarian exposition is nearly always not relevant.

Examining what we have discussed so far, it seems obvious that using the term 'clinical ethics' does not necessarily imply that one creates a new notion of medical ethics. At best it refers to the feeling that the common model of applied ethics needs amendment and revision. Clinical ethics itself is actually a borderline conception: it conveys new insights but it can easily be used to open up new contexts for the use of applied ethics without making these insights operational. In part, this is also the result of inadequate terminology: clinical ethics does indeed suggest only a new specific context, not a new conception of ethics adapted to all health care practices. In order to avoid the reduction of clinical ethics to applied ethics, we need a new term to make sure that we refer to a radically different self-interpretation of ethics.

5.2. Medicine and ethics as hermeneutics

Clinical ethics is a borderline case between applied ethics and a new conception of ethics, tentatively called hermeneutic ethics. Originally, *hermeneutics* referred to the art of interpreting and the science of interpretation. As such, it was used in theology, law and philosophy, all concerned with interpreting the meaning of texts. It has come into prominence in the last century as a methodology characterising the humanities and social sciences. Philosophers such as Schleiermacher and Dilthey have shown that not only texts but all human products need interpretation, and that hermeneutics involves not only the interpretandum but also the interpreter. Finally in our century, through the works of Heidegger, Gadamer and Ricoeur, hermeneutics evolved into a philosophy of understanding and explaining human existence.

Entering a new stage of the long-standing debate on the status of *medicine*, it has recently been argued that medicine has to be considered as a hermeneutical enterprise apparently presuming that medicine is not or not merely a natural science (Daniel, 1986; Leder, 1988). The modern emphasis on information and empirical data has contributed to new understanding of diagnosis and treatment as the physician's interpretation of what concerns the patient and what can be done to help the patient. And metaphorically, the patient is conceived as a text that may be considered on different interpretive levels.

It is important to reflect upon the typical preconditions of interpretation in medicine. The patient is usually understood through an anatomico-physiological model. The patient's body is made 'readable' by the use of technology. The biomedical language of diagnosis and treatment reduces the overwhelming amount of information presented by the patient so that the standard medical case report reflects not the story of the patient's life but of the physician's relationship with the patient's illness (Poirier and Brauner, 1988).

It is also important to look at the effects of medical interpretation upon the interpreter. Interpretation seems to bring understanding and empathy. Interpreting symptoms involves understanding what is actually wrong with a patient and appreciating what he or she is going through. Interpreting the patient's illness arouses therefore an 'affiliative feeling' in the physician–interpreter (Zaner, 1988).

Some contemporary philosophers have argued that *ethics* is best considered to be a hermeneutical discipline. As a particular branch of philosophy, ethics is proceeding from an empirical fund of knowledge, i.e. moral experience. The moral dimension of the world is first and foremost experienced. Moral experience is our way of understanding ourselves and or in the world in moral terms (Van Tongeren, 1988). Ethics is the interpretation and explanation of that primordial understanding. Before practising ethics we must already know, at least to some extent, what is morally desirable, obliged or right. Otherwise, we would not recognise what is appealing in a moral sense. But on the other hand, what we recognise in our experience is unclear and in need of elucidation and interpretation.

In short, we are approaching the moral dimension of the world from a set of prior understandings; they form the basis of our interest in what seems odd and strange to us, and what makes us reconstruct its meaning(s). Ethics therefore can be defined as the hermeneutics of moral experience.

5.3. Medical ethics as hermeneutics

The above ideas have occasionally been used to re-think conceptions of medical ethics. We can only offer a few programmatic thoughts upon a hermeneutic conception of medical ethics, summarising what seem to be its central characteristics.

1. *Experience*: The starting-point of medical activity is the moral experience of the patient. Through his illness he is confronted, in Zaner's (1988) words with tears in the fabric of daily life. He presents himself to the physician as both puzzling and meaningful. The patient's symptoms are deeply textured by his biographical situation, with his beliefs, values, habits and lifestyle. To ascertain what is wrong requires an interpretation, the more so since there is an initial distance between patient and physician. The meaning of the individual human being who is the patient requires interpretation for two reasons: firstly, intrinsic strangeness: the experience of illness in this particular patient is unique and unusual, and secondly, theoretical pre-understandings: the context in which the physician interprets the symptoms (e.g. the pathological models) is different from the context in which the interpretandum came into existence.
2. *Attitudes and emotions*: For ethics, the fundamental question is not so much 'What to do?' but rather 'How to live?' It is *praxis* not *poiesis* that is important (Van Tongeren, 1988). The moral relevance of our actions should not be reduced to their effects; it is also determined by an evaluation of what we do in executing our actions (for example, the problem of experimenting with human embryos should not be settled by reference to future results, but should also raise the question: Why are we interested in scientific research?). This change of focus implies a re-orientation from activity to passivity, from acts to attitudes and emotions. Moral experience involves primarily feelings, for instance, of indignation, confusion or contentment; secondarily, these emotional responses can be made the object of moral thinking (Callahan, 1988).

3. *Community*: The interpretive reading of a patient's situation is not an individual doctor's affair. The medical prior understandings that orientate the interpretation are the sediments of traditional cultural assumptions concerning the nature of the world and the body, and the results of a specific historical evolution of medical knowledge. Interpretation presupposes a universe of understanding. This is a consequence of the so-called hermeneutic circle; in order to interpret a text's meaning, the interpreter must be familiar with the vocabulary and grammar of the text and have some idea of what the text might mean (Daniel, 1986). For man as a social being, understanding is always a community phenomenon—understanding in communication with others. The continuous effort to reach consensus through a dialogue with patients, colleagues and other health professionals induces us to discover the particularities of our own prior understanding, and through that, to attain a more general level of understanding. This seems to reflect the experience of hospital ethics committees: analysing a case in terms of moral principles leads to a stalemate but interpreting the moral experience of the concrete participants involved in this particular case usually leads to a consensus.
4. *Ambiguity*: Hermeneutic ethics aims at interpreting and understanding moral experience. But moral experience is complex and versatile. It implies that every interpretation is tentative; it opens up a possible perspective. Definitive and comprehensive interpretation is non-existent. A hermeneutic approach always has an ambiguous status: more than one meaning is admitted. As Zaner (1988) points out: 'Every life is linguistically inexhaustible, there is always a richer tale to be told that can never be wholly captured in words, no matter how evocative they might be'. That means that moral judgments and decisions which must be framed on the basis of understanding the thematic moral ordering of a person's life are fundamentally uncertain.

   Because it is explicating the richness of moral experience, hermeneutic ethics may find itself making problems more complicated instead of providing clear-cut analyses and answers.

6. FUTURE CONSEQUENCES

6.1. A different practice of ethics

The hermeneutic conception has important consequences for the competence and role of medical ethicists. Since the interpretation of moral experience takes place within the context of particular social practices, intimate knowledge of the historical, medical and scientific components of those practices is essential to the task of moral criticism. Ethics cannot be practised without a high degree of engagement in medical work. Bedside medical ethics does not imply that only doctors can be ethicists. To comprehend the human terms in which actual moral dilemmas are experienced, the facts of medical practice must not be left to the doctors. But being able to do that requires a sharing of moral experiences of patients and doctors.

Understanding and defining the facts of the case do not involve the identification of relevant general principles and the deduction of a set of rules from which the correct response to the problem can be derived. The role of medical ethics is not so much to explicate and apply ethical theories and principles but to interpret and evoke what is implied in moral experience. The notion 'applied ethics' suggests wrongly that we already know which moral principles and rules to apply. However, rules and principles are in fact answers to what is evoked or appealed to in a particular case. First of all, we need to understand what the moral experience of vulnerability and appeal to assistance really means in this case. We need to discover why particular principles will motivate us in this case; why is there a particular ideal, rule or obligation? It requires close scrutiny of the medical situation in all its complexity. Only then will we recognise, as Noble (1982) emphasises, that 'the principles used to "justify" the social practices are only highly abstract descriptions of norms already embodied in those practices'.

6.2. Need of research

To implement the hermeneutic conception of medical ethics, more empirical study of actual decision making processes is necessary. Like the empirical turn in contemporary philosophy of science, research projects should combine medical sociology and anthropology, history of medicine and ethics to construct a more sophisticated view of moral experience in medicine. During the daily clinical work at a hospital medical department significant ethical problems were encountered in 25% of all patients (Kollemorten *et al.*, 1981); although a variety of ethical problems were identified, it was not clear how and why problems were labelled as moral problems.

A fine example of in situ research into the interpretation of moral experience is Bosk's (1979) study of the management of failure in a surgical service of a major American teaching hospital. He investigated the set of background understandings, norms, and values that are invoked to categorise clinical events as errors. By participant observation and interviews Bosk shows how the norms of clinical practice are constructed and learned during a surgical training programme; surgeons are frequently using tactics of interpretation to make a distinction between inevitable blameless failures and unforgivable errors, and within the last category, between technical errors and moral errors. It appears that moral errors are considered more serious than technical ones. Bosk relates this unexpected finding to the nature of the doctor–patient relationship and to the conspicuousness of moral performance in surgery. He concluded that 'postgraduate training of surgeons is above all things an ethical training'.

6.3. Clinical ethics teaching

If Bosk is right that the ethical dimensions of training are built into everyday clinical life, then the teaching of medical ethics should be concentrated in the clinical period. Hermeneutic ethics emerged from the now partly substantiated intuition that ethics is part and parcel of the routine practice of medicine, as well as from the feeling that ethics is not an abstract exercise of moral reasoning but characterised by the emotion, complexity and ambiguity commonly involved in real cases. These considerations have consequences for the method and goals of medical ethics teaching (Loewy, 1986; Ten Have and Essed, 1989). Preference should be given to team-teaching in the clinical period using the format of patient conferences and case review, generally accepted in routine clinical work. The objective of this problem-oriented ethics teaching is first and foremost to increase the students' sensitivity to moral problems in everyday medicine.

6.4. A new rapprochement between ethics and philosophical anthropology

During this century there seems to have existed an undercurrent of philosophical criticism of modern medicine with very different manifestations: originally scientistic, then anthropological, now ethical. It is striking that the philosophical–anthropological movement in Dutch and German medicine (represented by, for example, V. von Weizsäcker and F. Buytendijk) that was very influential from the 1930s, collapsed in the 1960s, at the time when interest in medical ethics was growing fast. The anthropological criticism with its strong moral undertones tried to re-orientate medicine from within and to reform it into a truly 'alternative' medicine (Ten Have, 1987). Our hypothesis, defended elsewhere, is that the recent success of medical ethics in its applied and analytical form has to be explained by its tendency to seek technical solutions for moral problems and to abstain from criticising the foundations of medicine (Ten Have and Kimsma, 1987). This success is bought at the price of an extraneous position, the reason why practising physicians may feel uncomfortable with applied medical ethics.

On the other hand, the hermeneutic conception of ethics argues that ethicists should not be observers but participants engaged in medical practice. It is remarkable that this conception also stimulates a renewed interest in philosophical–anthropological studies of the foundations of medicine.

Zaner's recent book illustrates the potential for a new encounter between ethics and anthropology (Zaner, 1988). Ethical discourse is incomplete without a phenomenology of illness and a philosophy of the clinical encounter. That is what physicians themselves used to do. Since moral experience is at the basis of good medical practice, and since good practice refers to philosophical ideas about the nature of medicine, they try to explicate that experience in an ideal of a good and competent professional.

REFERENCES

Beauchamp, T. L. and Childress, J. F. (1983) *Principles of Biomedical Ethics*, 2nd edn. Oxford University Press, New York, pp. ix–x.

Bosk, C. L. (1979) *Forgive and Remember. Managing Medical Failure.* University of Chicago Press, Chicago.

Brody, H. (1989) Transparency: Informed consent in primary care. *Hastings Center Report* **19**, 5–9.

Callahan, S. (1988) The role of emotion in ethical decision-making. *Hastings Center Report* **18**, 9–14.

Caplan, A. (1982) Applying morality to advances in biomedicine: can and should this be done? In: Bondeson, W. B. *et al.* (eds.) *New Knowledge in the Biomedical Sciences.* Reidel, Dordrecht, pp. 155–68.

Cassell, E. J. (1976) *The Healer's Art. A New Approach to the Doctor–Patient Relationship.* Lippincott, Philadelphia, p. 109.

Clouser, K. D. (1975) Medical ethics: some uses, abuses, and limitations. *New England Journal of Medicine* **293**, 384–7.

Daniel, S. L. (1986) The patient as text: a model of clinical hermeneutics. *Theoretical Medicine* **7**, 195–210.

Dworkin, G. (1988) *The Theory and Practice of Autonomy.* Cambridge University Press, Cambridge.

Ellul, J. (1954) *La Technique ou l'Enjeu du Siècle.* Armand Colin, Paris.

Greaves, D. (1979) What is Medicine? Towards a philosophical approach. *Journal of Medical Ethics* **5**, 29–32.

Heidegger, M. (1966) *Discourse on Thinking* (trans. J. M. Anderson and E. H. Freund). Harper & Row, New York, p. 51.

Heisenberg, W. (1971) *Schritte über Grenzen.* R. Pieper & Co., Munich.

Illich, I. (1975) *Medical Nemesis. The Expropriation of Health.* Calder & Boyars, London.

Jonsen, A. R. and Toulmin, S. (1988) *The Abuse of Casuistry. A History of Moral Reasoning.* University of California Press, Berkeley.

Jonsen, A. R., Siegler, M. and Winslade, W. J. (1986) *Clinical Ethics. A Practical Approach to Ethical Decisions in Clinical Medicine.* MacMillan, New York, p. 3.

Katz, J. (1984) *The Silent World of Doctor and Patient.* Free Press, New York.

Kierkegaard, S. (1978) Thoughts on crucial situations in human life. In: Oden, T. C. (ed.), *Parables of Kierkegaard.* Princeton University Press, Princeton, p. 38.

Kollemorten, I. *et al.* (1981) Ethical aspects of clinical decision-making. *Journal of Medical Ethics* **7**, 67–9.

Leder, D. (1988) The hermeneutic role of the consultation–liaison psychiatrist. *Journal of Medicine and Philosophy* **13**, 367–78.

Loewy, E. H. (1986) Teaching medical ethics to medical students. *Journal of Medical Education* **61**, 661–5.

Lyotard, J.-F. (1986) *La Postmoderne Expliqué aux Enfants*. Galilée, Paris.

Noble, C. N. (1982) Ethics and experts. *Hastings Center Report* **12**, 7–9.

Poirier, S. and Brauner, D. J. (1988) Ethics and the daily language of medical discourse. *Hastings Center Report* **18**, 5–9.

Ten Have, H. (1987) Afscheid van anthropologische geneeskunde? *Metamedica* **66**, 245–59.

Ten Have, H. and Essed, G. (1989) An experimental case-conference programme for obstetric and gynaecology clinical students. *Journal of Medical Ethics* **15**, 94–8.

Ten Have, H. and Kimsma, G. K. (1987) *Geneeskunde Tussen droom en Drama. Voortplanting, Ethiek en Vooruitgang*. Kok, Kampen.

Van Tongeren, P. (1988) Ethiek en praktijk. *Filosofie & Praktijk* **9**, 113–27.

Zaner, R. M. (1988) *Ethics and the Clinical Encounter*. Prentice Hall, Englewood Cliffs, NJ.

4

The Place of Values in Health Care: Recurring Themes in the Philosophy of Medicine

Ineke Widdershoven-Heerding, PhD

1. INTRODUCTION

In contemporary reflections on health care attention is being paid to the place of values in health care. Do values belong within the realm of the health professions or not? The answer to this question depends on the answer given to the question: 'Are dysfunctioning and disease value-free notions?'. Such concepts are fundamental to health care. All health professionals raise claims to be able to assist in preventing, alleviating and curing human dysfunctioning. One of the major efforts in the philosophy of medicine and the health sciences is therefore directed at clarifying these concepts.

The value-ladenness of human dysfunctioning has been contested most in the aspect of bodily dysfunctioning. Is it justified to maintain that somatic disease is a normative concept? And, consequently, have those health sciences that deal with somatic disease necessarily an ethical component? The solution to this problem, whether disease is a value-free notion or not, has given rise to much discussion in contemporary philosophy of medicine.

The ethical responsibility of health care professionals remains unclear, as long as the place of values, and of ethical decisions, in health care seems undefined. Are health care professionals scientifically trained experts possessing knowledge of human functioning which they may or may not apply, depending on the request of the autonomous patient? Or is the application of their knowledge inherently justified by their assessment of the patient? In the first case their professional activity should be

---

Changing Values in Medical and Health Care Decision Making
Edited by U. J. Jensen and G. Mooney

supplemented by external ethical elements; in the second case their activity may in itself be called normative. The diagnosis is internally related to notions of solidarity and concern for the suffering and distress of others.

The current argument for and against a morally neutral, objectivistic definition of disease is not entirely new. At the turn of the century the question whether disease is a value-free notion or not was widely discussed. A description and analysis of this historical debate may help us to clarify some aspects of the contemporary discussion. The historical review of several difficulties associated with a scientific conception of medicine will perhaps unveil some implicit assumptions and also some weak spots in the modern scientific concept of health care. It may also shed new light on the differences between individualistic and social autonomy.

2. HISTORICAL PERSPECTIVE

When we place the historical debate about the place of values in health care in its context, we must realize that this debate 80 years ago centred around the question of whether medicine was a value-free enterprise or not. At the end of the 19th century the scientific status of medicine seemed established. Since the 1840s medicine has been put forth as a science by such well known authors as Schwann (1910), Virchow (1847, 1975), Naunyn (1869), du Bois-Reymond (1891) and von Helmholtz (1903) and in Holland by, for example, Donders (1971) (see also Rothschuh, 1978). They all claimed that medicine should be included among such sciences as physics and chemistry.

Medicine was to be a purely empirical science, employing experimental methods and aiming at scientific understanding, i.e. an explanation, in terms of chemical and physical laws, of disease. Organic and inorganic nature were considered equal in scientific research; the same methods and procedures were applied (cf. Galaty, 1974). Non-scientific notions were totally banished from medicine. Vitalism and teleology were rejected, but also ethical views and metaphysical assumptions were put aside as not belonging within the realm of medicine (e.g. Donders, 1971). Medicine as a science should be value-free, and any intrinsic connection with values seemed a contamination of the scientific character of medicine. Medicine thus conceived as an empirical science is necessarily associated with a scientific conception of disease. In contrast with former notions, specifically of the *Naturhistorische Schule*, one of the tenets of scientific medicine is that disease is a process. In 1869 Virchow defined it thus: 'Die Krankheit ist ein Lebensvorgang, überhaupt nicht ein Wesen, sondern ein Vorgang, der durch eine gewisse Sukzession von Zuständen verläuft, von denen der eine mit einer gewissen Notwendigkeit aus der anderen hervorgeht'. (Virchow, 1975).

Disease processes are life processes, reconstructed scientifically as causal sequences and governed by physical and chemical laws. Disease processes do not differ qualitatively from other processes in life. From a scientific perspective on life we find mechanical functioning everywhere and, in this respect, health and disease are alike and as such indiscernible (see Donders, 1971). In the second half of the 19th century it was felt necessary to stress this point over and over again because of the danger of relapsing into an ontological concept of disease, one of the major faults of former medical thought.

Virchow declared in 1847 that: 'Krankheiten nur den Ablauf der Lebenserscheinungen unter veränderten Bedingungen darstellen'. Consequently it is the task of medicine to produce 'die normalen Bedingungen des Lebens'. Virchow uses here the word 'normal' in an empirical sense without ethical implications.

Changed life conditions result in cellular changes and changed cellular processes. These latter processes form the core of Virchow's concept of disease. Cellular processes are, as everything else, ruled by chemical and physical laws. Virchow hoped to uncover these in his pathophysiology. Pathophysiology would provide those trained in it with the tools to explain and manipulate disease processes. Material circumstances cause disease and an analysis of this process indicates, in principle, how and when the doctor can intervene. Even a calculation of the outcome of the medical intervention seems possible on the basis of the pathophysiological laws. One of the major claims of scientific medicine in those days was that it offered perspectives in therapy.

A noteworthy presupposition of the scientific conception of medicine is that it is based on human equality. As human beings we are all prone to suffer from the same disease in the same circumstances. Physical and chemical laws apply to everyone, without distinction. And as human beings are only relevant to scientific medicine at the level of their material functioning, it seems reasonable to dispel such value-laden and perhaps undemocratic notions as constitution and disposition from medicine. They only confuse and obscure the real purpose of medicine—the causal explanation and treatment of disease following empirical, experimental methods. The old-fashioned paternalistic country doctor without a sophisticated scientific training is outdated compared to those trained in objective medical science.

The concept of human equality is also one of Virchow's arguments in favour of a social medicine. According to Virchow it is possible, statistically, to discover which part of the population is threatened most with disease and early death. In some sections of the population the conditions of life are worse than in other sections. It is the task of medicine to ameliorate these circumstances, to provide normal conditions for life. When the poor suffer more often from disease, this cannot be explained indifferently by their specific constitution. Medicine has social and political implications; hence Virchow's well known thesis, 'medicine is a social science'. The notion of human equality, a presupposition of scientific medicine, led Virchow to social involvement.

This essential feature of scientific medicine, human equality in the face of disease, is most clearly expressed in the views of one of the two most prominent forms of scientific medicine at the end of the last century, the bacteriological school of Koch, Klebs *et al.* As opposed to Virchow, they state that it is much more useful in medicine to search for external causes of disease, instead of unravelling cellular processes. With Koch's discoveries the optimism grows that one day it will be possible to identify one external factor, a parasitical micro-organism, as *the* cause of a specific disease.

The monocausal hypothesis of the bacteriological school falls clearly within the range of scientific medicine, as the adherents of the bacteriological school repeatedly claim. Methodological materialism, one of the corner-stones of scientific medicine, remains totally unchallenged. Moreover the bacteriologists work according to empirical standards and follow experimental methods.

Virchow is nevertheless sceptical in 1895. According to him the bacteriologists tend to confuse the cause of disease with the disease process itself. They seem to fall into ontological traps. Whereas Virchow emphasized that health and disease differ only in degree, they are both subsumed under the term life, the bacteriologists draw a sharp demarcation line. The presence of parasitical micro-organisms is equated with disease; the absence of such micro-organisms with health. Virchow, and within a decade many others, pointed to the fact that, though disease processes often start following some intrusion from a parasitical micro-organism, they do not necessarily occur (Virchow, 1895). The presence of specific micro-organisms is not a sufficient condition for disease processes.

The bacteriological school unintentionally made one point clear: human beings are unequal with respect to their bodily functioning. The same parasitical agent does not trigger the same disease process in each individual human being. The prediction of human functioning appears to be more complicated than the bacteriologists, and also Helmholtz and other prominents of scientific medicine, expected (Virchow, 1877; von Helmholtz, 1903; Bernard, 1957). Medicine deals with objects more complex than the scientific conception of medicine initially assumed. Empirical tests proved not to be such unequivocal and adequate standards as had been hoped.

At the turn of the century, following the period of the bacteriologists' monocausal optimism, much attention was again paid to the individual properties of organisms. The former wisdom in medical practice, that every patient reacts differently to the same influences, no longer seemed an old-fashioned unscientific rule of thumb. Concepts such as disposition and constitution regain importance in medical thinking.

Circa 1900 the energetistic school of Rosenbach, Hueppe and Martius tried to reconcile concepts such as constitution and disposition with scientific medicine (Hueppe, 1923; Martius, 1923; Diepgen, 1926). They criticized the bacteriologists because of their one-sidedness in pathogenetic questions. They rejected the idea that bacilli are the only and sufficient cause of disease. The energetistic school drew attention to the well known observation that the nature and the external conditions of a stricken organism also play their role in the development of diseases (cf. Martius, 1923).

The energetistic conception of medicine was inspired by Mayer's (1952) law of the conservation of energy. The adherents of the energetistic school were impressed by the conjunction of what at first sight appeared such divergent qualities, by reducing them to energy. They proposed to apply this same procedure to the different factors in the human constitution. In the individual constitution, biological and social factors, hereditary qualities and cytological qualities are all summed together. These factors serve as a latent condition to the occurrence of disease. Constitution is qualified as potential energy. The actual disease is caused as a result of this equilibrium of energy being disturbed. The energetistic approach in medicine thus reduces pathological factors to different amounts of energy. Pathology has become a sort of calculus. Disease is, according to Hueppe (1923), a function of disposition, external conditions and an instance, e.g. a microparasite which actualizes the tensile force. Life is an ongoing exchange of energy and all individual differences are translated into specific amounts of energy.

In the energetistic attempt to combine a purely quantitative perspective with medicine, one of the fundamental issues in medicine seems to have disappeared. In the continuous flow of energy it is impossible to discern healthy from diseased. Graul (1917), following Martius, defines disease thus: 'stets ist Krankheit der Ausdruck funktioneller Disharmonien nach irgendeiner Richtung hin'. But how can we discover whether *dis*harmonies take place? And is the presence of disharmonies sufficient cause to apply the notion disease?

In its quest for scientific rationality, medical thinking seems to have lost sight of its basic concepts. Lubarsch, a prominent German medical author and editor in the first decades of this century, pointed out in 1917 that medicine is not served by Martius's reasoning. When Martius claims that man is the cause of disease or that life is the cause of death, this has no special value for medicine. Both are necessary conditions, certainly, but they are not relevant to medicine. Lubarsch endorses Virchow's view that disease is only gradually and not essentially different from health. Nevertheless, medicine is interested in precisely those circumstances that bring about disease and death. Relations between different quantities of energy can therefore never provide a basis for medicine.

The period following the scientific era in medical thinking shows a renewed interest in the difference between organic and inorganic nature. Metaphysical notions like teleology are no longer banished (Mayer, 1952). To comprehend disease it is considered necessary to understand the harmony in nature, which is essentially more than material mechanical functioning. The organistic era in medicine tries to relate medicine again to certain norms and values. Scientific analysis is supplemented by teleological reasoning. Though the organistic solution is not very satisfying from our contemporary point of view, it is born from a genuine concern, the impossibility of medicine as a value-free science.

3. CURRENT THINKING

Today medicine claims to be a science again. Of course our conception of science differs from the classical concept of the 19th century. Nevertheless we perceive certain resemblances, especially when we direct our attention to the modern concept of disease, or human bodily dysfunctioning. In both conceptions of science, values are placed outside the realm of science. So, human dysfunctioning as a scientific concept has no normative component. Human dysfunctioning is to be measured objectively, by comparing actual functioning to biological norms.

The contemporary scientific definition of disease has been presented by Boorse (1977): 'A disease is a type of internal state which is either an impairment of normal functional ability, i.e. a reduction of one or more functional abilities below typical efficiency, or a limitation on functional ability caused by environmental agents.' He contends that his conception of disease requires no value judgment about what forms of human life are admirable or desirable. Eliminating disease, the task of the health care professional, is, according to Boorse, uniquely describable in advance of normative decisions.

Boorse's conceptions of disease and of the activities of the health care professional seem to echo Virchow's opinions. Medical science has no need for an ethical component. Morally good health care consists of the application of medical techniques for the correct purposes. Medical experts possess knowledge and an individual may claim their assistance when he or she is in need. Modern health care professionals are able to estimate the different outcomes of different treatments. In medical decision analysis experts are able to sum quantitatively many divergent aspects of the individual situation, the goal of the energetistic school. And in the ideal situation it is up to the patient to decide which treatment will be chosen. The scientific conception of disease as the objective, non-normative account of the facts concerning the functioning of an individual human being then leads easily to the adoption of the principle of deontological autonomy.

The scientific conception of disease is not unchallenged. Engelhardt (1975, 1986) and Whitbeck (1981), and formerly King (1954), propound that disease is a value-laden concept. This normative view propounds that the conception 'disease' is fundamentally associated with human valuation. Disease is not primarily a deviation from the species norm, but it is first and foremost an undesired situation. Disease prevents people doing the things that people in their circumstances commonly do. Diseases interfere with our body and, more generally, with our well-being. Moreover, disease elicits therapeutic action and support (cf. Miller Brown, 1985).

The normative approach stresses the differences between human biology and medicine, or between the basic sciences and clinical medicine. The equating of scientific statistical norms with health and disease is rejected. While the latter are always placed in a societal context, they are related to human cultural standards. The normative conception of disease relates the suffering of the individual not only to the deviation from objective standards but also to shared values. King (1954) defines disease thus: 'Disease is the aggregate of those conditions which, judged by the prevailing culture are deemed painful, or disabling and which, at the same time, deviate from either the statistical norm or from some idealized status'. Human dysfunctioning can only be understood within a social context. This normative component explains the sympathy and concern for the diseased, expressed by their fellow-beings.

Jensen and Mooney contend, in their introduction to this book, that the basic moral principle of responsibility for the weak ought to be one of the basic values in the health care system. This ethical principle of solidarity leads them to a plea in favour of the adoption of the principle of social autonomy in health care. The arguments of Jensen and Mooney are mainly concerned with the macrolevel of organization and distribution in health care systems. From the historical debate we may also draw some arguments in favour of a normative conception of disease and consequently in favour of a notion of social autonomy, on the level of clinical practice. Clinical judgment, as the assessment of disease, and clinical practice are incomprehensible without reference to values. The nature of clinical judgment requires a more encompassing concept of autonomy than the individualistic conceptions of autonomy connected with the scientific concept of medicine.

REFERENCES

Bernard, C. (1957) *An Introduction to the Study of Experimental Medicine*. Dover Publications, New York.

Boorse, C. (1977) Health as a theoretical concept. *Philosophy of Science* **44**, 542–73.

Caplan, A. L., *et al.* (eds) (1981) *Concepts of Health and Disease. Interdisciplinary Perspectives*. Addison-Wesley, Massachusetts.
Diepgen, P. (1926) Krankheitswesen und Krankheitsursache in der spekulativen Pathologie des 19. Jahrhunderts. *Archiv für Geschichte der Medizin* **XVIII**, 302–27.
Donders, F. C. (1971) *De Harmonie van het Dierlijke Leven. De Openbaring van Wetten*. Oosthoek, Utrecht. pp. 9–12.
du Bois-Reymond, E. (1891) *Ueber die Grenzen des Naturerkennens, Zwei Vorträge von Emil du Bois-Reymond*. Leipzig.
Engelhardt Jr, H. T. (1975) The concepts of health and disease. In: Engelhardt Jr, H. T. and Spicker, S. F. (eds) *Evaluation and Explanation in the Biomedical Sciences*, Reidel, Dordrecht, pp. 125–41.
Engelhardt, Jr, H. T. (1986) Clinical complaints and the *ens morbi*. *Journal of Medicine and Philosophy* **11**, 207–14.
Engelhardt Jr, H. T. and Spicker, S. F. (eds) (1975) *Evaluation and Explanation in the Biomedical Sciences*. Reidel, Dordrecht.
Galaty, D. H. (1974) The philosophical basis of mid-nineteenth century German reductionism. *Journal of the History of Medicine* **29**, 295–316.
Graul, G. (1917) Ueber die Erkenntnis des Krankheitsgeschehens. *Deutsche medizinische Wochenschreibe* **43**, 1541–2, 1567–8.
Hueppe, F. (1923) Ergographie. In: Grote, L. R. (ed.) *Die Medizin der Gegenwart in Selbstdarstellungen*, Leipzig, p. 16.
King, L. (1954) What is disease? *Philosophy of Science* **21**, 193–203.
Lubarsch, O. (1917) Ueber Aufgaben und Ziele der pathologischen Forschung und Lehre. *Deutsche medizinische Wochenschreibe* **43**, 1377–80.
Martius, F. (1923) Autoergographie. In: Grote, L. R. (ed.) *Die Medizin der Gegenwart in Selbstdarstellungen*, Leipzig, p. 24.
Mayer, C. F. (1952) Metaphysical trends in modern pathology, *Bulletin of Historical Medicine* **XXVI**, 71–81.
Miller Brown, C. (1985) On defining 'disease'. *Journal of Medicine and Philosophy* **10**, 311–28.
Naunyn, B. (1869) Antrittsvorlesung, Dorpat.
Rothschuh, K. E. (Hrsg.) (1975) *Was is Krankheit?* Wissenschaftliche Buchgeseelschaft, Darmstadt.
Rothschuh, K. E. (1978) *Konzepte der Medizin in Vergangenheit und Gegenwart*. Hippokrates, Stuttgart, pp. 417–47.
Schwann, Th. (1910) *Mikroskopische Untersuchungen über die Uebereinstimmung in der Struktur und dem Wachstume der Tieren und Pflanzen*. Leipzig.
Virchow, R. (1847) Ueber die Standpunkte in der wissenschaftliche Medicin. *Archiv für pathologische Anatomie und Physiologie und für klinische Medicin* **I**, 3–19.
Virchow, R. (1877) Ueber die Standpunkte in der wissenschaftliche Medicin. *Archiv für pathologische Anatomie und Physiologie und für klinische Medicin* **LXX**, 1–10.
Virchow, R. (1895) *Hundert Jahre allgemeiner Pathologie*. Berlin, p. 38.
Virchow, R. (1975) Ueber die heutige Stellung der Pathologie. In: Rothschuh, K. E. (ed.) *Was is Krankheit?* Wissenschaftliche Buchgeseelschaft, Darmstadt, p. 85.
von Helmholtz, H. (1903) *Das Denken in der Medizin. Vorträge und Reden*, Vols 1 and 2. Friedrich Vieweg, Braunschweig, p. 183.
Whitbeck, C. (1981) A theory of health. In: Caplan, A. L. *et al.* (eds) *Concepts of Health and Disease. Interdisciplinary Perspectives*. Addison-Wesley, Massachusetts.

5

Building Networks: A Constructivist Perspective on Changes in Medicine and Health Care

G. L. Wackers, MD

1. INTRODUCTION

Modern medicine and health care have changed rapidly in almost every aspect during recent decades. The body of medical knowledge has increased considerably. We have witnessed the emergence of a wide array of new technologies for research, diagnosis and therapy. The costs of health care have risen. Economic constraints have become visible and social and political attitudes towards medicine and health care have shifted.

These changes in knowledge, technologies, values and socioeconomic structures, etc. have taken place simultaneously and are dependent on one another. Once this is agreed it becomes impossible to discuss them separately, for example looking at cognitive or technological changes separately from changes in moral values.

In philosophies of science and in ethics or moral philosophy distinctions between internal scientific developments and external social influences, between content and context, facts and values, have long been cherished and maintained. These philosophical distinctions give rise to different and basically asymmetrical explanations. Concepts like rationality, reality and laws of nature are used to explain progress and success in science, whilst morality is grounded in the social, in notions about human nature or in some religious authority. The inadequacy of these 'purifying' accounts is exposed when they are confronted with the impurity of scientific and medical practices.

Changing Values in Medical and Health Care Decision Making
Edited by U. J. Jensen and G. Mooney

Recent work in the field of social studies of science and technology tries to overcome the distinctions between content and context, between science and technology on the one hand and society on the other. In section 2, I will outline briefly some characteristic trends in the type of analysis attempted in these studies. In the remainder of this chapter I will, firstly, introduce one of the theories in this area of research, the *actor–network theory* developed by Callon *et al.* (1986) and Latour (1987) and secondly, try to extend this approach from science and technology to moral values, in an attempt to account for concurrent changes in knowledge, technologies and values in modern medicine and health care in a single analytical endeavour.

In section 3, I will use a brief account of the 'discovery' of insulin as an example to illustrate the notion of *building or constructing a network*. This account enables us to grasp some important features of scientific and technological change which have a significant bearing on an understanding of the role and fate of moral values in health care. These features will be presented in more detail in sections 4 (on black-boxing), 5 (on heterogeneous engineering), and 6 (introducing the notion of translation), using contemporary examples in sections 5 and 6. Sections 7 and 8 deal with the emergence of controversies, introducing the concepts of direction of movement and of spokespersons. Section 9 emphasizes the importance of the stabilization of a network and the creation of a private space to avoid the interference of opponents. Finally, in section 10 I will explore the consequences of this approach for our understanding of moral values, their change, force and durability.

2. A NEW TYPE OF STUDY ON SCIENCE AND TECHNOLOGY

The publication of Kuhn's *Structure of Scientific Revolutions* in 1962 is said to mark a historical turn in the study of science. Since the 1970s students of science, technology and society have made a sociological turn. Detailed empirical studies of historical and contemporary scientific and technological developments are used as a starting point for theoretical reflections on science and technology. The burden of centuries of positivist philosophy and Whiggish history writing was shaken off. Distinctions between science, technology, economics and society do not exist 'out there'. They are constructed by philosophers of science, devoting their time to the design of philosophical schemes to explain the rational growth of knowledge; by economists studying the impact of technological developments on the economy; and by sociologists studying the impact of science and technology on society. It is in their work that distinctions between pure and applied research, between internal developments and external influences arise. It is in like manner in the work of historians that the Great Men of science emerge, men who bring about entire revolutions on their own. It is only when we assume that our current knowledge is the truth that we can look back in time and distinguish between those who were right and those who were wrong.

The sort of analysis attempted by those taking the sociological turn is characterized by three trends:

1. They move away from the great, individual inventor or scientist as an *explanatory* concept.
2. They do away with, or deconstruct, the old divisions and employ the metaphor of a *seamless web* to express that these traditional distinctions do not help us to understand what science and technology is about or how it works.
3. They emphasize that our analysis should be *symmetrical*: we should be able to explain both the success and the failure of facts and artefacts with the same theoretical concepts (Bijker *et al.*, 1987). We should not, in other words, resort to reality when explaining successful theories and technologies, and to ideologies and interests to explain the failures. There is a basic notion behind this requirement: the way we conceive reality is the result of the closure of scientific controversies, and cannot be used to explain the closure itself or the success of the 'victor'.

Within this field three different approaches can be distinguished, which differ in the theoretical concepts used:

1. A systems approach stemming largely from the work of the historian of technology Thomas Hughes.
2. The social constructivist approach developed by Bijker and Pinch, inspired by recent studies in the sociology of scientific knowledge.
3. The actor–network theory, which will be introduced in the sections which follow.

3. BUILDING A NETWORK

The metaphor of a network is used to emphasize that modern medicine is a very heterogeneous structure in which different kinds of elements are associated together (physicians, patients, hospitals, diagnostic and therapeutic technologies, pharmaceutical companies supplying drugs, health insurance companies, regulatory laws, medical faculties, research programmes and so on). The elements in the network are interdependent. Their identity is determined by their mutual relationships. A stabilized network both shapes and supports its elements. The notion of a network is best understood when we look at the work that has to be done to build one. Let us take an example from the history of diabetes mellitus: the 'discovery' of insulin[1]. This provides us with a general overview over a longer period of time. In the next sections contemporary examples are used to show in more detail what constructing a network entails.

Insulin is now used by millions of diabetic patients to regulate their carbohydrate metabolism. It is produced by pharmaceutical companies and brought to the patients through an almost worldwide distribution network. This was not so a century ago. In 1889 insulin did not exist. Diabetes mellitus did exist and resulted in the deaths of many patients. Physicians had not much to offer. The notion of internal secretion was coined in 1855 by Bernard, but it did not have the same meaning as we attribute to it today. The pancreas was known to secrete digestive juices into the gut, having no relationship to diabetes mellitus[2].

In 1889 Minkowski succeeded in performing a total pancreatectomy on a dog[3]. This dog became diabetic. So did several other dogs on which he operated. For Minkowski this was a strong indication that the pancreas was involved in diabetes mellitus in humans.

The research conducted on this subject in subsequent decades by Minkowski, Hédon, Zuelzer, Opie and several others can be characterized as:

1. explaining why other researchers doing pancreatectomies on dogs did not report their animals becoming diabetic. By scrutinizing these reports, Minkowski showed that in all animals at autopsy there was a small remnant of pancreatic tissue left.
2. establishing a strong link between the pancreas and diabetes. Minkowski's experiments did not convince everybody. Several investigators produced alternative explanations for the increased excretion of sugar in the pancreatectomized dogs.
3. showing that diabetes mellitus was not linked to the known exocrine secretion of the pancreas. Hédon did important work, both to strengthen the link between the pancreas as a whole and diabetes, and to weaken the link between the exocrine secretory function of the pancreas and the disease. In the first stage of his operation he took out almost all of the pancreas, completely and irrevocably cutting off the supply of pancreatic juice to the gut. He left a small remnant of pancreas, still nourished by

1. A detailed constructivist account of this discovery will be published elsewhere.
2. There were some reports in which diabetic patients at autopsy were shown to have abnormal pancreases. This link between the pancreas and the diabetes was as weak—or as strong—as the link between the liver or the stomach and diabetes.
3. The first total pancreatectomy performed by Minkowski was not an endocrinological experiment. It was a demonstration to Von Mehring, who was doing research into the role of the pancreas in the digestion of food in the gut, that it could be done.

its blood supply and pulled it out through the wound and grafted it under the dog's skin. The dog did not become diabetic. But when Hédon completed the pancreatectomy by cutting off the blood supply to the remnant of the graft, diabetes immediately developed.

4. establishing a link between diabetes and the islands of Langerhans, known as a histological entity but with unknown function. Eugene Opie linked pathological changes in Langerhans' islands and diabetes. Langerhans' islands provided a good candidate for the site of production of 'the active principle regulating carbohydrate metabolism'. In other words, they provided an anatomical substratum for the hypothetical endocrine function of the pancreas.
5. making a pancreatic extract that was able to lower the blood sugar level in diabetics without giving toxic reactions. Many investigators recognized that the best evidence for the internal secretion theory of the origin of diabetes would be an antidiabetic effect of a pancreatic preparation, administered parenterally. The absence of toxic reactions was important because these kept alive the alternative explanation that the decrease in the output of sugar was the result of a toxic or depressor action, and not of a specific regulatory action of the pancreatic secretion.

It can hardly be said that insulin, and as a consequence the very endocrine function of the pancreas, really existed between 1889 and 1921. In spite of the 'strong theoretical inducements' derived from Hédon's experiments, the record of the search for insulin is a record of failure. Frederick Allan, known for his work on the *Total Dietary Regulation in the Treatment of Diabetes* (1919), wrote in 1913: 'All authorities are agreed upon the failure of pancreatic opotherapy in diabetes. Injections of pancreatic preparations have proved both useless and harmful. The failure began with Minkowski and has continued to the present without an interruption. The negative reports have been numerous and trustworthy'. The dilemma in which these scientists found themselves is expressed by Macleod in his book *Diabetes: Its Pathological Physiology*, published in 1913. After due deliberation he concluded that there was an internal secretion of the pancreas, but he suggested at the same time that it might never be captured in a pancreatic extract. This 'scientific' dilemma resolves or closes *after* the stabilization of insulin in 1921.

In 1921 in Macleod's laboratory in Toronto, Canada, Frederick Banting and Charles Best performed the experiments for which Banting and Macleod were awarded the Nobel Prize for medicine, late in 1923. They 'discovered' insulin.

Why were they successful where others failed? Was Banting a brilliant experimenter, a genius, as hagiographic history writers would want us to believe? Did he have brilliant ideas?

On the contrary, Banting, being a young surgeon in 1921, was a newcomer to the field of experimental research on diabetes mellitus and carbohydrate metabolism. Charles Best was a young science student assigned to him by Macleod to do the chemical tests necessary for the work. They made the same 'mistakes' as other scientists in the field before them had done.

The difference was in the 'shape of the network' they established: their collaboration with Collip, a chemist with experience in protein chemistry and the co-operation with Eli Lilly and Company, brought in to help prepare the pancreas extract in commercial quantities. This company established the links with slaughterhouses that had to supply beef and pork pancreases. It helped the scientists to beat off challenges to Toronto's priority and to win the battle on patents on pancreas extracts. The Toronto Insulin Committee was set up to standardize the extracts and to control and distribute the licences to produce insulin in other countries (Bliss, 1982).

In the Netherlands, the Dutch licensee Ernst Laqueur, professor in pharmacology at the University of Amsterdam, persuaded Saal van Zwanenberg, director of Zwanenberg's Slachterijen en Fabrieken (Zwanenberg's Slaughterhouses and Factories), to form a new pharmaceutical company: Organon[4].

The pancreas with its islands of Langerhans is as much an element in this network as insulin itself is. So are the pharmaceutical companies producing it, the physicians prescribing and the patients using it.

It is important to notice that many of these elements are transformed in the process of their enrolment into the network. The stabilization of the network, after a period of more than 30 years, redefines the identity of the pancreas into an endocrine gland. Langerhans islands, left without a definite function since their establishment in 1869, are finally equipped with one in 1921. Zwanenberg's Slachterijen en Fabrieken is transformed into Organon. The disease, diabetes mellitus itself, is redefined as an endocrine metabolic disorder. The balance of power between the disease on the one hand and the physician and the patient on the other is inverted, thereby profoundly changing the management of diabetic patients in clinical practice[5].

4. Organon is the Dutch pharmaceutical company known for the production of hormones. Insulin was the first drug produced by Organon. Laqueur moved his laboratory to Oss and became head of Organon's research laboratory. See Tausk, M. (1978) *Organon. De Geschiedenis van een Bijzondere Nerderlandse Onderneming*. Dekker & Van de Vegt, Nijmegen.

5. In subsequent years new elements have been transformed and assimilated into this network. In the 1970s *Escherichia coli* is transformed by means of recombinant DNA techniques and is now producing large quantities of human insulin in barrels. See Hall, S. (1987) *Invisible Frontiers. The Race to Synthesize a Human Gene*. Atlantic Monthly Press, New York.

The brush used to paint this picture of building a network is too crude, and the strokes are too coarse to discern the role and fate of values in this process. We should at this point resist the temptation to assign to one basic value, for example to combat death and prolong life, the power to guide a large group of physicians and scientists in their search for an effective treatment for diabetes mellitus. Yet, this rather crude description of part of the history of diabetes mellitus and insulin does enable us to grasp some significant features of scientific and technological change. The discussion of these features in the next sections can shed new light on our understanding of moral values.

4. BLACK-BOXING: FROM HYPOTHESIS TO RESOURCE

An important feature of scientific and technological change, demonstrated in the history of insulin, is the transition of a hypothesis into a resource. Between 1889 and 1921 the existence of an active principle regulating carbohydrate metabolism, the endocrine function of the pancreas and the involvement of Langerhans' islands were all hypothetical. Nobody could take them as given. After 1921 the situation was radically different. Insulin turned from a hypothesis into a resource that could be bought from Eli Lilly and Company and from Organon and deployed to combat a lethal disease. This transition process is called *black-boxing*. Black boxes are facts and artefacts that can be taken for granted. In other words, the factual status of knowledge and technologies that are black-boxed is—or is claimed to be—beyond dispute (Latour and Woolgar, 1986).

Black-boxing is accompanied by some secondary processes in which, retrospectively, disputes about priority are settled and credit for the 'discovery' is attributed. Another important secondary process is the elimination, in writing and talking, of all traces of the construction of a fact or an artefact. Allusion to any hypothetical or theoretical status of a fact is gradually eliminated from scientific texts. What once was a hypothesis, insulin, is now an entity in the world.

Another example can perhaps emphasize this point even better. We all know now that cells are the functional units that constitute our body. At the beginning of the 19th century the scientific literature was imbued with allusions to the *Schwannian* cell *theory*, the validity of which remained to be settled. Cells are black boxes now.

It is important to stress here that black-boxing cannot be explained by referring to some intrinsic quality of a scientific statement or a technology, or to reality or laws of nature. Black-boxing is the result of the actions others exert on a statement or technology: scientists accepting and reinforcing the claim, using it as established knowledge in their subsequent research; physicians using a technology as a resource in the treatment of patients.

The black-boxing of facts and artefacts and the stabilization of relationships between these elements enables physicians in day-to-day medical practice to take short-cuts. A physician can diagnose a case of diabetes mellitus on the basis of a blood sugar level that is over 11 mmol/l, taken 2 hours after a meal rich in carbohydrates. He or she can refrain from measuring insulin concentrations in blood and from histological examination of pancreatic tissue. He or she can take a short-cut between the blood sugar estimate and the syringe with insulin bought from Eli Lilly.

Thus far we have considered an example where the movement was in a positive direction: from hypothesis to fact, technology and stabilized network, serving as a resource for physicians and patients. The brief account of the history of insulin in section 3 also reveals that over a number of years things tended to move in the opposite direction, that the hypothesis about the endocrine secretion of the pancreas was likely to turn out to be false.

The very *fate*, positive or negative, of the work of scientists or engineers—of network-builders in general—fact or artefact, is in the hands of others (Latour, 1987). It may be grasped, heralded, considered a major breakthrough, worthy of an award—maybe even the Nobel Prize. Or it may be repudiated, considered to be simply false or fraudulent, a threat to humanity. This dependence of knowledge claims and technologies on the actions that other people exert on it is what makes building or extending a network so difficult. An attempt to establish new or better knowledge, or to improve existing technologies and procedures may even fail in the initial stage of a research proposal or a grant application. A contemporary example can illustrate this, simultaneously allowing the discussion of another important feature of scientific and technological change: the heterogeneous character of the work, and the heterogeneity of the elements associated together in arguments and networks.

5. HETEROGENEOUS ENGINEERING

Geraedts, a Dutch scientist currently working in the field of anthropogenetics and cell biology at the University of Limburg, is participating in the in vitro fertilization (IVF) programme in Maastricht. He wants to produce new and better knowledge about the initial stages of development of the human embryo, about the effects of freezing on the ovum and the early stages of development after fertilization. He wants to evaluate the safety of new microtechniques through which sperms are directly injected into the ovum and to improve the success of IVF and embryo transfer (ET)[6].

6. Microinjection techniques are intended as a therapy for male infertility.

Geraedts designed a research programme to address some of these questions. Because the clinical IVF programme of the hospital yields too few 'spare' embryos to do the research, his proposal involved the utilization of human embryos produced in the laboratory for this purpose—the embryos not used for therapeutic purposes are considered to be of lesser quality on morphological grounds.

Geraedt's grant application was successful in getting the research financed. However, he did not get the approval of the institutional review board (IRB) and the board of the hospital. Human embryonic life should not be used in a purely instrumental way. Geraedts had to direct his efforts through animal research.

At the same time however he joined forces with an ethicist, De Wert, and published a co-authored article on 'IVF, pre-embryo research and ethics' (De Wert and Geraedts, 1988). This article contains a string of arguments in which methodological and empirical claims are mixed with cognitive, philosophical and ethical arguments. The authors introduce the notion of a pre-embryo to indicate the stages of development during the first 2 weeks after the fertilization of the oocyte, in accordance with existing conventions in human embryology—based on morphological criteria—to designate this period as blastogenesis. They tie this notion to the philosophical concept of a person and argue that a pre-embryo is not yet a person, but has the potential of becoming one. The degree to which the early stages of human life deserve protection depends on the degree to which this potential is realized. The Kantian imperative that human life should never be used in an instrumental way cannot be maintained in an absolute sense.

The authors carefully juxtapose several black boxes in their string of arguments. Established black-boxed knowledge about human embryos is gratefully taken for granted and used to build a strong argument. They also use a specific philosophical concept of a person as a black box. At the same time they try to open and devalue the black boxes of their opponents. They strengthen their own case by mobilizing Tejada and Karow through a citation. These authors state that 'not withstanding the heated debate between the pro-life and the pro-choice groups, the descriptive morphologist, the embryologist, and the IVF practitioner must be guided by what *the microscope shows,* regardless of criticism by *nonscientific discipline'* (my emphasis; Tejada and Karow, 1986).

A few months later new actors entered the stage, being neither scientists nor ethicists. The moral status of human embryos in research appeared on the programme of a symposium organized to mark the publication of a new Dutch textbook on medical ethics. De Wert, a contributor to the book, defended his position there. The symposium attracted the attention of the media. Several national newspapers, radio stations and television programmes devoted space and time to the planned research by Geraedts on human embryos. This publicity transformed the matter into a political issue. For different reasons spokesmen for the political parties opposed this kind of research stating that they would explicitly ban it in a forthcoming bill concerned with experiments on human beings. Politicians and administrators thus linked their judgment about the value of beginning human life to a legal framework to strengthen its position and contribute to its black-boxing, that is, to its status as an indisputable value in itself.

Geraedts is now likely to be confronted with a legal ban on research on human embryos produced for non-therapeutic purposes. He failed to establish a necessary link with the IRB and to control the actions exerted by journalists and politicians on his proposals.

How can we conceptualize the networking of elements as heterogeneous as the ones described above in relations to one another which are equally heterogeneous? How and why do controversies about the moral or legal status of human embryos or zygotes arise in the first place? To tackle this problem we have to introduce the concept of *translation*.

6. TRANSLATION

In a general sense, translation stands for all the mechanisms and strategies through which one actor identifies other actors and elements and places them each in relation to one another (Callon *et al.*, 1986). The concept of translation covers two important aspects of the processes we try to understand. It refers to *transformation* (change of identity) and to *displacement* (movement, change of place).

The pancreas was transformed into an endocrine gland and placed in a strong relationship with diabetes mellitus. Diabetes itself was transformed and displaced. From 'out there', where it killed many patients and could not be managed, it was moved to the laboratory where it could be manipulated, transformed and conquered. Zwanenberg's Slachterijen en Fabrieken was transformed into a pharmaceutical company. Laqueur literally moved his equipment from his laboratory in Amsterdam to Organon in Oss to set up Organon's first research laboratory.

Translation pertains not only to the transformation and displacement of things, people or companies. It also accounts for shifts in *problem definitions, solutions* and *responsibilities*. An infertile couple, who want to have a child *of their own*, have to move their problem to the expert's office, into a network that may offer a solution. They may have to revise their definition of the problem to accommodate it to whatever it is that the network has to offer, and transform what counts as a solution to their problem, for example when artificial insemination by donor semen or adoption are the only options left to them. The 'of-their-own' part of both the problem definition and the solution has to be omitted (de Vries, 1988).

The gynaecologist harvesting the oocytes from a woman's ovaries through a laparoscopic operation moves them to the laboratory where they can be fertilized. But it is not just the cells and the fertilization process that are moved to the laboratory. With them, the responsibility for what happens to them—both in a technical and in a moral sense—is also translated to the laboratory.

It is through these translations that new situations and new problems arise. The question of what is to be done with embryos that are not re-implanted in a womb arises only after the oocytes are translated to the laboratory. Should we flush them down the drain, or use them in experimental research? Or should we freeze them and use them later when the first attempt to establish a pregnancy has failed, because we hold that these embryos should at least be given a chance to realize their potential of becoming a human being? Must we, thinking along these lines, allow re-implantation into a woman who is not the donor of the oocyte? Who is the mother in such a situation?

Scientific, technical, moral and legal problems arise simultaneously. Traditionally unproblematical notions about who the mother is become problematical and have to be renegotiated, as a result of which new words are added to the dictionary. Questions about what constitutes a person, about the circumstances under which human life deserves utmost respect and protection, and about the conditions under which instrumental use is allowed or forbidden have to be settled. Several social groups are involved in this process and none of science, philosophy, or ethics determines the outcome.

Along the same lines we can account for controversies about the value of life in another area—quality versus quantity of life—and about definitions of death with accompanying criteria. The use of resuscitation techniques, of artificial respiration and circulation supporting technologies, in many cases displaces death from the patient's side. They enable physicians to keep patients alive and stabilize their condition. The heart–lung machine makes it possible to bypass the heart entirely and to operate on people, take their heart out and implant a new one.

However, death is not the only one who is displaced. Responsibilities are translated too. Multiple problems arise simultaneously. What is the value of life when the patient's condition stabilizes at a low level? Is it worth living? What has to be done with patients who stay in a persistent vegetative state for many years? Are they to be kept alive or should we 'pull the plug'? Who decides on these questions?

When should death be pronounced? What criteria have to be fulfilled to call *some-body* a corpse? When are we allowed to extirpate organs for transplantation? Is it equally unacceptable, from a moral point of view, to treat the dead as if they were living as it is to treat the living as if they were dead (Veatch, 1976)?

Goals of health care have to be renegotiated. Fixing malfunctioning mechanisms and prolonging life at all costs are no longer the overriding goal of health care. The quality of life has to be taken into account too.

Death has to be redefined. Cessation of the heart beat doesn't suffice any more. This becomes strikingly apparent when we look at the short period of time during a heart transplantation when the patient's heart is taken out and the new heart is not yet implanted.

Redefining death is not just a diagnostic problem, which can be solved by science. It is closely related to philosophical and moral notions. Like participants in the discussion about the moral status of human embryos, participants in the negotiations about definitions of death employ different *problem definitions*.

Articulating a particular problem definition can be seen as an actor's attempt to translate other actors, one of the mechanisms by which actors try to build and extend their own network. In general, problem definitions involve a *dual mechanism*. First of all an initial frontier is traced between what is analysed and what is not, between what is considered relevant and what is suppressed, kept silent. It carves out a territory, cut off from the outside. Next, within this domain a second frontier is traced between what is considered irrefutable, firmly established and what is problematical or unknown (Callon, 1980). Articulation of a research problem must necessarily be founded on established knowledge, methods, previous studies and basic assumptions.

Geraedts's definition of his research problem traced a specific frontier between the unknown that has to be studied on the one hand—the teratogenic effect of freezing and thawing on human embryos—and the unproblematical on the other—the moral status of the cells with which he would be working. The IRB traced another frontier, thereby casting doubt on what Geraedts considered unproblematical.

A problem definition offered may be accepted or rejected by others. Others can force us to employ another problem definition. Problem definitions with different degrees of generality may be linked together. A general problem definition pertaining to controlling the rising costs of health care, formulated by health care authorities, may be readily accommodated and linked to a more specific problem definition concerning the relative benefit of IVF over alternative options to treat infertility (microsurgery of the fallopian tubes), adopted by a university's health economics department. The latter problem definition can in turn be accommodated to the problem of designing computer software for cost–benefit calculations in a mathematics department.

The clinical problem of treating infertility can be linked to specific biological problems about the nutritional or chemical conditions under which fertilization of the oocyte occurs.

In other words, general problem definitions are translated into more specific ones and moved to other institutions or to another level in a hierarchy. Through the successful *networking* of problem definitions the initial frontiers traced are basically retained and reinforced.

It may be apparent from these examples that nobody builds a network in empty space. Other actors are building or managing other networks. There is an uninterrupted process of translation and counter-translation going on, generating tensions, conflicts and struggles. According to Callon *et al.* (1986), this continuous process leads to:

1. The fixation of the identity of actors, their interests and their strategies, being always temporary.
2. The definition and 'networking' of problems.
3. The objectification, remodelling and transfer of knowledge.
4. The establishment of hierarchies between organizations, groups and individuals.

7. DIRECTION OF MOVEMENT

Conflicts do not always arise. They are most likely to emerge when people try to do different things, reach different goals, adhere to different values. Conflicts will not appear when actors move in the same direction (Latour, 1988).

A patient in a diabetic coma sliding away into death, an empty-handed physician, and a scientist offering an experimental pancreas extract shown to decrease the excretion of sugar in five diabetic dogs, were moving in the same direction. Banting and Eli Lilly and Company were moving in the same direction. So were Laqueur and Saal van Zwanenberg as they joined forces and founded Organon. A cell-biologist doing research on the early stages of human development moves in the same direction as the gynaecologists responsible for the IVF programme. An ethicist can join the team when he also moves in the same direction. Infertile couples desperately wanting a baby move in the same direction as the physicians building an IVF network. In a public debate, defending the IVF programme against criticism about high costs and low success rate, physicians are likely to argue for the patient's autonomy, her constitutional right to health care and the physician's moral and professional obligation to help those who come to him for help.

Physicians who do not want to comply with requests for voluntary euthanasia—on moral or religious grounds or because they are afraid of the legal consequences—are *not* moving in the same direction as their patients asking for help. They declare themselves to be morally obliged *not* to assent to the patient's request. Now it is the patient, or somebody who speaks for him, or her, who has to claim the individual's autonomy in these matters. Geraedts and the IRB did not move in the same direction, although they did not come into frontal collision. The IRB did not deny the importance of the research. They might even have granted their approval when only spare human embryos were involved.

By taking the direction of movement of different actors into account we can understand the vehement protest of the Dutch gay movement against Swaab's statement that in 15 gay men who died of acquired immune deficiency syndrome (AIDS), the suprachiasmatic nucleus in the brain was distinctly larger than in heterosexual men or females[7]. Swaab is a neurobiologist working at the Brain Institute in Amsterdam. He is doing research on AIDS-related changes in the brain. In particular he is interested in the question of whether the dementia seen in AIDS patients, which in many respects resembles Alzheimer's dementia, is associated with the same anatomical changes in the brain. In Alzheimer's disease the suprachiasmatic nucleus undergoes degenerative changes and becomes smaller. His research revealed that the suprachiasmatic nucleus was enlarged in 15 gay men who died of AIDS. Comparison with the brain tissue of heterosexual men who died of AIDS revealed that the enlargement of the nucleus was not AIDS-related. Swaab did not say in his public statement that the enlarged nucleus causes homosexuality. He simply stated an objective fact, a coincidental finding, a byproduct of his research.

Nevertheless, a storm of protest raged through the public media. Questions were asked in Parliament. Swaab was accused of being naïve and inconsiderate, of not seeing the risk of an upsurge of discriminating activities against homosexuals and misuse of this kind of information. He was accused of breaching the trust of these patients, who before they died gave their informed consent to the research. However the consent was given to investigate the causes of AIDS and not the causes of the patient's homosexual disposition. In terms of science policy it was said that this kind of research should be given lowest priority. There are many other more urgent questions to which scarce resources could be allocated. Nobody disputed the 'objective fact' of the enlarged suprachiasmatic nuclei. Nobody said: 'Show me your slides. I don't believe you'. Spokesmen for the gay movement traced entirely different frontiers in their definition of the problem. They have been moving for many years in the opposite direction.

The vehemence of the protest can only be understood if we take into consideration that the gay movement has been striving to get homosexuality out of the World Health Organization classification of diseases, to get it out of medical and psychiatric textbooks where it was labelled as a sexual

7. This account is based on the public discussion in newspapers etc. in January 1989.

perversity. Any attempt to establish or even suggest a link between any anatomical difference or physiological disturbance and homosexuality will be counteracted[8]. The gay movement tried to raise a road-block for Swaab, they tried to displace him.

8. SPEAKING FOR THE MUTE

There is another concept—already implicit in the examples given thus far—that can improve our understanding of changes in values in medicine and health care and the emergence of controversies. That is the notion of a *spokesperson*.

In ordinary parlance political parties and unions have spokesmen or women. They are supposed to speak for a group of people, members or voters. These people could speak for themselves, but they delegate this task to one who speaks for them all. In court we have a lawyer who speaks for us. We could speak for ourselves if these legal matters were not so complicated that it takes an expert to speak for us.

In medicine many patients can speak for themselves, but there are important categories who cannot, because they are *mute*. Embryos and pre-embryos are mute. They cannot speak up to protest when they are flushed down the drain, or when their cell divisions are interrupted to assess their chromosomal constitution. Comatose patients are mute. They cannot object when the plug is pulled. But they cannot object either when it is not. The mute have to be spoken for.

A wide array of spokespersons speak for the mute: physicians, nurses, relatives, ethicists, theologians, politicians, the state. The pro-life movement also speaks for the mute. Spokespersons move, so to speak, in front of the mute. They translate themselves into the mouthpiece of those who cannot speak.

But not only the mute are spoken for. We also speak for the ignorant: the mentally retarded, the disabled, the insane. There are also spokespersons for the un- or less-educated. In fact every patient, every individual—patient or not—is spoken for nowadays. Of course, it is possible to distinguish between competence and capability regarding the expression of will in those spoken for, but this does not change the essence of what spokespersons do, speaking *for* others.

In recent decades we have witnessed the emergence of a multitude of professional and institutionalized spokespersons, people who studied

8. It is interesting to see that a professor in *transsexuality* welcomes any research that could lead to new possibilities to *cure* transsexuals.

philosophy or law, now working in university departments or in the service of interest groups. It is what they do for a living. They know about constitutional rights, moral theory and philosophy. They translate philosophical and moral notions into the string of arguments they are building. They know how to speak, how to write and how to behave in the public arena to win over their audience. They sail a collision course if necessary.

As a result of their activity the freedom of movement for scientists and physicians is reduced; in other words, the frontier between what may be called the public and the private space is displaced, renegotiated.

9. STABILIZATION

It is here where the importance of the notion of *stabilization of a network* becomes apparent. Doing research and treating patients would be impossible if everything were renegotiable at any time, if at any time anyone could move in and object to what we are doing. One important result of successful heterogeneous engineering is the creation of a stable and private space—at least for a set period. A private domain appears when our work is paid for and material requisites are available, when we can get the approval of the IRB if required, and when our work fulfils relevant legal requirements. In this private domain we can pursue our business, not at will, but relatively sheltered.

The outside world, the public domain, becomes less important. Not every objection is *relevant* any more. Or, expressed in a more 'pregnant' way: when legal, financial and human actors (physicians, patients) sustain a practice of contraception or abortion, it does not matter that the Pope does not agree.

The stabilization of a network creates a *horizon of relevance* between the inside and the outside. Actors within this horizon do not have to negotiate any more about problem definitions, established knowledge or basic values, not as long as the established horizon of relevance is successfully managed.

10. VALUES REVISITED: STRENGTH FROM WEAKNESS

Let us now try to harvest what we have been sowing in the preceding sections. How does all this bear on our understanding of moral values and their change?

Many values appeared in the examples given, most explicitly when there was a controversy. We saw the value of prolonging life and combating untimely death in the case of diabetes mellitus. We saw how the absolute value of beginning human life, following from the Kantian imperative, was relativized to improve the technique of IVF and ET, which in turn was said to pursue the fulfilment of other values: the patient's autonomy, the constitutional right to health care or the value of having children. We also saw how beginning human life was protected against instrumental use. The value of the quality of life and of dying came forward simultaneously with an appeal to the patient's autonomy in the light of the technological means to sustain circulation of blood and respiration artificially. In the case of the gay movement's protest against Swaab's findings, autonomy concerning sexual preferences and the notion of informed consent appeared side by side with the value of non-discrimination.

Value judgments never appeared alone. They were always linked with other elements—cognitive, technological, legal or philosophical—to build an argument as strong as possible, frequently to serve another goal. Apparently some strength can be derived from value judgments that merit their explicit enrolment into a string of arguments. Apparently values serve as a resource that can be handled as a black box.

Black boxes tend to be devoid of traces of their construction, at least when they are not contested. The source of their strength that makes them stand as a self-evident, self-containing truth is however revealed when they are challenged, when they are *tried by disagreement* (Latour, 1988). The physician questioned about his short-cut between a blood sugar estimate and the syringe with insulin, in other words for his taken-for-granted reliance on these black boxes, will show us his medical textbooks and the work done by Minkowski, Banting, Best and many others as a reply. If we wished to disagree with Swaab's statement about the size of the suprachiasmatic nucleus he would show us the slides of brain tissue from homo- and heterosexual men and females, the atlas on the anatomy of the brain and the manual of the microscope to convince us of the quality of its measuring device. If we were going to challenge established embryological knowledge, Geraedts would mobilize embryologists, microscopes and slides of human embryos. It is from these sources that black boxes derive their power.

The questions to be asked now are these: From what or whom do moral values derive their strength? Who or what is mobilized when a moral value is called in for assistance?

Uffe Juul Jensen gives us a hint when he discusses the responsibility for the weak as a basic moral principle (Jensen, 1987). Jensen conceives of values as 'model activities or paradigmatic examples of responsible action and ethical importance, serving the role of models and paradigms in ordinary human life . . . We are acting morally responsibly towards other individuals or groups who in a particular context are weaker than us, if we try to act from their point of view, and support them'.

The *weak* are mobilized when values are invoked. Values gather strength from the weakness of the innumerable patients who died from infectious diseases and from other diseases like diabetes mellitus. Statistics are not important here. It is the repeated personal experience of empty-handed, powerless physicians that counts. Values derive their strength from the weakness of beginning human life not allowed to develop its potential of becoming a human being, sucked away in artificially induced abortion or simply flushed down the drain. Strength is gained from the weakness of those who are not allowed to die but are kept alive in a persistent vegetative condition, from the weakness of the dead who are treated as if they were living. Strength is gathered from the weakness of those who are denied a job, battered or killed for the colour of their skin, for their sexual preference or for their religion.

The weak are mobilized when values are invoked. This is not just another metaphor. They are mobilized when these values are violated or challenged. Many of the weak are dead or hidden from view. They have been overpowered. But some of them leave traces that remind us of their struggle: diaries, pictures, films, written records and case reports, names engraved in memorial stones. Remnants of the second world war's concentration camps, Anne Frank's diary and war cemeteries fulfil the same functions as Amsterdam's gay monument, pictures of mutilated embryos and fetuses, and case reports on patients who are in a coma for many years. It is through these traces that the weak are mobilized. But what are they mobilized for, and by whom?

The weak of the past are mobilized to mobilize the living—IRBs, politicians, the legislator, public opinion—to protect today's and the future's weak. They are mobilized by people who speak in the name of yesterday's weak on behalf of the weak of the present.

Jensen judges this speaking for and acting on behalf of the weak morally responsible when it is pursued from the perspective of the weak and aims at their support, at a reduction of inequality, not only between individuals but also between individuals or groups on the one hand and society or lifeforms on the other. This kind of model activity is present in our everyday life and has been present throughout history.

But what makes it a *model* activity, a *paradigmatic example*, of morally responsible behaviour to be used by people as a *standard* for commenting on and judging past and future actions? Jensen seeks the answer in the nature of human communal life: human beings living in relationships with others, characterized by dependence and power. It is in the establishment of these relationships that the moral responsibility for other individuals or groups, who are weaker than us, is established.

Our analysis suggests another answer. There is nothing in the activities of people exhibiting solidarity with the weak that makes us necessarily perceive these actions as good or morally responsible. Neither do we possess some kind of moral sense organ in our human psychophysiological constitution. Instead of looking for some quality in the activity itself, in human nature or in the nature of human relationships, we have to look at *subsequent* actions of others. The fate of value judgments is equally dependent on the actions of others as the fate of facts and artefacts. If we agree on the inclusion of poetry and literature in the notion of artefact, Barbara Hernstein Smith's observations on the *value of 'great poetry'* can serve to emphasize this point: 'The recommendation of value represented by the repeated inclusion of a particular work in anthologies of "great poetry" not only promotes but goes some distance of *creating* the value of that work, as does its repeated appearance on reading lists or its frequent citation or quotation by professors, scholars, critics, poets and other elders of the tribe; for all these acts have the effect of drawing the work into the orbit of attention of potential readers and by making the work more likely to be experienced at all, they make it more likely to be experienced as valuable' (Hernstein Smith, 1988). Thus, the reason why Jensen's model activities stand out as paradigmatic examples of morally responsible behaviour lies in the agency of spokespersons, including himself, who point them out as such. It is their repeated recommendation of these model activities as good—among other things in writing and teaching—that contributes to their status as a yardstick and their pursuit by others. Spokespersons add to and amplify the strength derived from the weak themselves, thereby translating a moral judgment from an instance of 'just giving public vent to private preferences' into a 'social force' capable of changing established practices.

The mobilization of the weak and of living allies is not sufficient to create *durability* or *obduracy* of values. It may turn out to be a brightly flickering flame of moral indignation, burning itself out after some time when the spread of flames does not result in the establishment of new practices, new ways of doing things. It is the incorporation in practices that makes values durable and obdurate. Established practices can be conceived as stabilized networks comprising a private space where physicians, patients and scientists can pursue their goals. Within these established practices new technologies are developed. Medical practices concerned with the treatment of lethal diseases developed techniques for artificial respiration, resuscitation and intensive care. Practices dealing with infertility problems developed techniques for IVF and ET. New problems arose in these practices through the pursuit of their goals. They created a new class of *new weak*. These new weak were and are spoken for. Spokespersons mobilized allies to protect them and to change existing practices or establish new ones, to establish new ways of handling comatose or incurably ill patients, new ways of handling beginning human life.

The shape of these new practices, these new networks, depends on the balance of forces involved, who is enrolled by whom, who resists enrolment into the network of others. New practices may supersede old ones, or they may emerge alongside pre-existing practices. Values are integral elements of and in medical practices. Their force is confined to these practices. They do not float around through empty space. They cannot be imposed on other practices, not without doing the work necessary to change these networks.

REFERENCES

Allan, F. (1913) *Studies Concerning Glycosuria and Diabetes*. Cambridge, Massachusetts.

Allan, F. M., Stillman, E. and Fitz, R. (1919) *Total Dietary Regulation in the Treatment of Diabetes*. New York.

Bernard, C. (1855) *Leçons de Physiologie Expérimentale Appliquée à la Médecine*. J. B. Baillière, Paris.

Bijker, W., Hughes, T. and Pinch, T. (eds) (1987) *The Social Construction of Technological Systems. New Directions in the Sociology and History of Technology*. MIT Press, Cambridge, Massachusetts.

Bliss, M. (1982) *The Discovery of Insulin*. University of Chicago Press, Chicago.

Callon, M. (1980) Struggles and negotiations to define what is problematic and what is not. The socio-logic of translation. In: Knor, K. D., Krohn, R. and Whitley, R. (eds) *The Social Process of Scientific Investigation*. Reidel Publishing, Dordrecht.

Callon, M., Law, J. and Rip, A. (eds) (1986) *Mapping the Dynamics of Science and Technology. Sociology of Science in the Real World*. Macmillan Press, London.

De Vries, G. (1989) Ethische theorieën en de ontwikkeling van medische technologie. *Kennis en Methode* **XIII**, 3, 278–94.

De Wert, G. and Geraedts, J. (1988) IVF, pre-embryo-research en ethiek. *Metamedica* **67**, 106–23.

Hernstein Smith, B. (1988) *Contingencies of Value. Alternative Perspectives for Critical Theory*. Harvard University Press, Cambridge, Massachusetts.

Jensen, U. J. (1987) *Practice and Progress. A Theory for the Modern Health Care System*. Blackwell Scientific Publications, Oxford.

Kuhn, T. (1962) *The Structure of Scientific Revolutions*. University of Chicago Press, Chicago.

Latour, B. (1987) *Science in Action. How to Follow Scientists and Engineers through Society*. Open University Press, Milton Keynes.

Latour, B. (1988) *The Pasteurization of France. Irreductions*. Harvard University Press, Cambridge, MA.

Latour, B. and Woolgar, S. (1986) *Laboratory Life. The Construction of Scientific Facts*. Princeton University Press, Princeton.

Macleod, J. J. R. (1913) *Diabetes: Its Pathological Physiology*. London, New York.

Tejada, R: J. and Karow, W. G. (1986) Semantics used in the nomenclature of IVF, or let's all be more proper. *Journal of In Vitro Fertilization and Embryo Transfer* **3**, 341–2.

Veatch, R. (1976) *Death, Dying and the Biological Revolution. Our Last Quest for Responsibility*. Yale University Press, New Haven.

6

Medical Decision Analysis and the Coming Moral Crisis in Health Care

R. J. Verkes, MD and P. J. Thung, MD

1. INTRODUCTION

Over several decades now, anxiety about modern medicine and health care has been brewing in most western countries. The roots of this unrest are manifold, but they are mostly related to imbalances between the span and power of medical science and technology on the one hand and the restrictions and imperfections of medical practice on the other. In practice, physicians choose from an ever-growing array of diagnostic and therapeutic procedures on the basis of habit or convenience rather than after weighing carefully all possible options and outcomes. Defensive medicine and sloppy routines are cases in point, implying overinvestment of means and efforts in relation to actual gains, or underinvestment vis-à-vis what could have been gained. Other imbalances occur where medical diagnosis and treatment do not correspond with the patient's perception of the problem or his or her expectations. Examples are paternalistic medicine and neglect of the communicative part of medical practice. Imbalances between cure and care also come under this heading: disproportional medical zeal may be focused on the disease process, to the neglect of what can and should be done for the general well-being and comfort of the patient. Last but not least, social inequalities in health care should be mentioned. Both nationally and internationally, imbalances occur between what medicine can and should do for society and what is actually available for large sections of the population.

Here we will not review these issues, some of which are discussed in the introductory chapter to this volume. For a general introduction and further

Changing Values in Medical and Health Care Decision Making
Edited by U. J. Jensen and G. Mooney

references see van der Steen and Thung (1988). It will be clear, however, that throughout these discussions moral values are at stake. Imbalances between means and ends, disagreement between problems as defined medically and as perceived by patients, and inequity in the provision of health care all depend on what values are considered relevant and how they are weighed. Medical effectiveness may seem a technical matter but turns into a moral issue when weighed against patient preferences. The issue of mere survival versus quality of life is a case in point. Similarly, investments in health care are not a purely financial question. The interests of providers and consumers lend a moral dimension to this as to all economic matters. This chapter starts from the observation that problems, like the ones signalled above, have kindled an acute interest in medical ethics. During the last 20 to 30 years, ethical teaching and research programmes have been started in many medical faculties. Journals and societies concerned with ethics in medicine have been founded. Ethical assessment procedures are increasingly being introduced in hospitals and research institutions. In our opinion, a process of 'rethinking medicine', in terms of the morality of its means and ends, is under way and will, within the next few decades, reshape the medical landscape.

However, ethical revival has not been the only reaction to imbalances in medicine and health care. Some 10 years ago, a new discipline was introduced to medicine with the recommendation that it could help to sort out and solve those problems arising because of the luxuriant growth and complexity of medical data and options. Medical decision analysis (MDA) offered techniques for systematizing and rationalizing processes of choice and decision under conditions of uncertainty inherent to most medical actions. Decision analysis can be traced back to the early 1940s when Von Neumann and Morgenstern (1944) published their *Theory of Games and Economic Behaviour*. It was not until the late 1960s, however, that it developed into an independent discipline and began to shop around for opportunities of application. It first became established in the field of business administration, but around 1980 medical applications of decision analysis were well developed and claimed the attention of clinicians and health service planning agencies (Pliskin and Pliskin, 1980; Weinstein and Fineberg, 1980). Its message can be summarized as follows:

1. MDA can implement systematic *feedback* from the wealth of medical research findings to medical practice. At the same time, it reveals areas of ignorance and uncertainty, thus indicating directions for further research.
2. It clarifies and structures discussions about medical decisions. The issues at stake are more clearly *explicated*, rendering the process of weighing and choosing more efficient.

3. MDA also helps towards distinct allocation of *responsibilities*. This is most relevant where decisions are taken under conditions of scarcity or where interdisciplinary co-operation is required.
4. It moreover opens the way for accommodating *individual* patient characteristics and value preferences in complex decision problems.
5. In general, MDA furthers *rational* and *systematic* procedures of decision making.

It should be noted, however, that MDA has so far found little acceptance in medical practice. Few practitioners are enthusiasts of MDA and most research in the area is done by statisticians and others not actively engaged in medicine. The impact of MDA on the Dutch medical literature has recently been analysed by Warndorff *et al.* (1988). Reviewing five volumes (1982–1986) of nine Dutch medical periodicals, they found 38 papers (out of 6750) on MDA. The majority of these (27) discussed the pros and cons of MDA. Only three papers demonstrated actual use of MDA for solving a medical problem. Arguments against MDA dominated in five papers (eight were more or less neutral; 14 papers were mainly in favour of MDA). These arguments ranged from intuitive aversion (MDA kills creativity, is incompatible with live doctor–patient interaction, etc.) to simple misunderstanding (MDA restricts freedom of choice, is expensive). The authors conclude that the impact of MDA on Dutch medicine is as yet negligible. In our opinion, the method seems to go against the grain of some notions and habits cherished by clinicians. Not only is it fairly time-consuming, but it also has little regard for personal clinical experience since it always prefers documented data over intuitive opinions.

Moreover, MDA emphasizes the need to quantify factors which are usually conceived in qualitative terms only. This is most relevant when medical decisions have to take account of personal preferences and values. MDA here advocates explicit and quantitative approaches which fit badly with the intuitions of doctors as well as those of patients. This issue may well turn out to be the acid test of MDA. In our opinion, MDA will in the future gain medical acceptance only if it can solve at least some of the problems raised in the moral debate about medicine and health care. In the next section we will tentatively explore one of the issues involved—the concept of quality-adjusted life years.

2. QUALITY-ADJUSTED LIFE YEARS (QALYs)

'Quality of life' is a concept which was introduced to medicine in the 1960s when it became increasingly clear that modern medicine often procures survival at very high prices in terms of harmful side-effects, pain, invalidity or other forms of suffering. For a review of early literature we refer to Najman and Levine (1981). What concerns us here is the way in which MDA tries to take into account qualitative aspects of survival in the course of rational and systematic decision analysis.

In MDA the relative desirabilities of possible outcomes of alternative treatment strategies are represented unidimensionally by quantitative 'utilities'. The concept of quality-adjusted life years (QALYs) has been designed in order to combine duration and quality of survival on one dimension. The use of QALYs as a decision criterion is based on three assumptions (Pliskin *et al.*, 1980):

1. Life expectancy (years) and health status (quality) are mutually utility-independent. This means that the form of the utility function over life expectancy does not depend on the particular level of health status, or the other way round.
2. There is a constant proportional trade-off between life expectancy and health status. The proportion of remaining life years that one is willing to give up for a specific improvement in health status does not depend on the absolute number of remaining life years involved. Suppose for example that an individual, in order to experience an improvement from 'moderate pain' to being 'pain-free', would be willing to sacrifice 3 of his remaining 15 years of life expectancy, i.e. 20%. If the constant proportional trade-off assumption applies, then this individual, if faced with a remaining life span of 20 years, would sacrifice the same proportion, i.e. 4 years, to achieve the same improvement in health status.
3. The third assumption deals with individual risk behaviour and will not be discussed in this chapter.

The question now arises whether the theoretical assumptions required by MDA make any sense in relation to human reality. How valid are notions like utility-independence and constant proportional trade-off in actual medical practice? It is clear that in at least some cases they are not valid at all. As shown by Sutherland *et al.* (1982), patients who are very ill may conceive a notion of a maximum time span beyond which they cannot endure their condition. Within this 'maximum endurable time' a proportional trade-off may more or less obtain, but survival beyond this time span carries a negligible or zero value. At that point, such patients would trade 10 more years in their present condition for 1 day of good health.

A similar observation was made by McNeil *et al.* (1981) when asking healthy subjects about their preferences when they were afflicted with laryngeal cancer. Would they choose laryngectomy, with high survival expectancy, or a more conservative treatment with lower survival but without losing the faculty of normal speech? Most subjects seemed willing to trade some years of survival for maintenance of normal speech, provided their expected survival was 25 years or more. However, if fewer than 5 years of survival were foreseen, few would sacrifice any of these for maintenance of normal speech. Thus their behaviour in choosing showed neither utility-independence nor trade-off constancy.

It would seem that MDA's use of QALYs, if at all valid, is practicable mainly under conditions of relatively good health states and long survival expectancies. Originally, however, decision problems involving serious impairment of health and brief survival were the main reason for introducing the concept of quality of life. Other problems with QALYs, as discussed by Mooney (1989), also suggest that this concept may be a supportive but hardly a sufficient tool for solving problems of medical choice under conditions of real life.

3. OTHER DUBIOUS ASPECTS OF MDA PROCEDURES

Figure 6.1 exemplifies the kind of decision problem to which MDA applies. There is a choice of alternative actions ($A_1, A_2 \ldots A_n$) with possible consequences or outcomes ($C_1, C_2 \ldots C_m$). In these outcomes, different parameters may be combined (e.g. duration and quality of survival) and to each outcome a quantitative utility can be assigned. Thus the expected utility can be calculated for each action, i.e. the weighted (for probability) average utility of the action in case. The optimal action or action of choice is the one with the highest expected utility. This criterion is known as the maximum expected utility (MEU). Assuming that the decision tree is an adequate

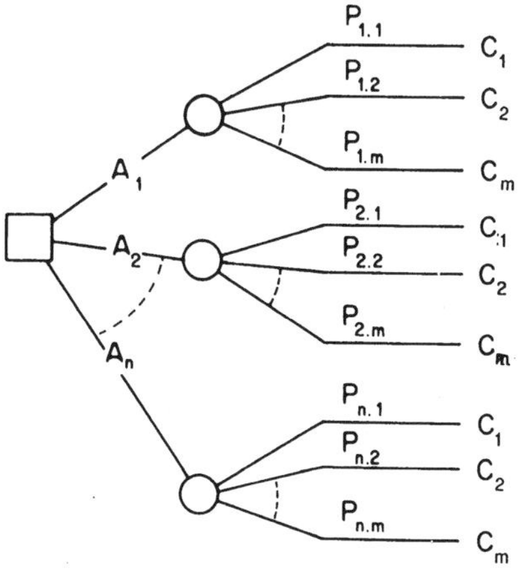

Figure 6.1 Model of a decision tree, showing alternative actions $A_1, A_2, \ldots A_n$, each with possible consequences or outcomes $C_1, C_2, \ldots C_m$. $P_{1.1}, P_{1.2}, \ldots P_{n.m}$ indicate probabilities of various outcomes. For further explanation see text.

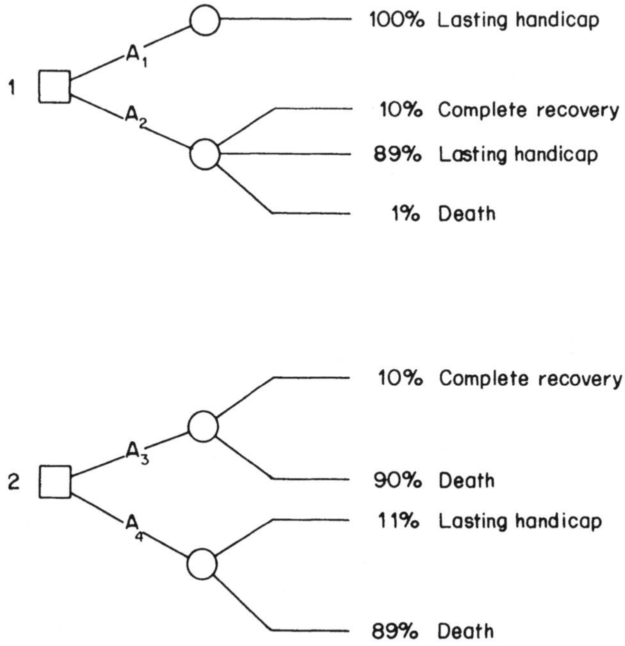

Figure 6.2 Two decision situations, in a modification of the Allais paradox (see text).

representation of the problem, then MDA theory posits that the MEU-carrying alternative is the only rational choice of action. This aspect of MDA theory, however, entails the following paradox. Figure 6.2 shows two related decision problems, i.e. starting from two different preoperative health conditions but involving similar therapeutic procedures. The figure is in fact a modification of the so-called Allais paradox (after the 1988 Nobel prize winner for economics). In both cases the patient may survive but with different chances of perfect recovery, depending on the action chosen. When confronted with the alternatives in each of these two situations, one might easily choose A_1 and A_3 respectively. In the first situation the 1% probability of death in option A_2 is disagreeable. In the second situation one may perceive the chances of death as practically equal and therefore opt for a chance of complete recovery by choosing A_3. A combined preference for A_1 and A_3 therefore seems acceptable.

This combination, however, is not justifiable according to the MEU criterion. In decision analysis, utilities are assigned to outcome independent of the probabilities. In both situations, the utilities of the outcomes therefore are identical. It is easily calculated that if A_1 carries the highest *expected* utility, then A_3 does not carry the MEU in the second situation and vice versa.

This paradox can be explained in terms of anticipated regret or rejoicing. Regret may be defined as the painful recognition that 'what is' compares unfavourably with 'what might have been' (Sugden, 1985). Conversely, if 'what is' compares favourably with 'what might have been', one will experience pleasure which may be called rejoicing. In the first situation of Figure 6.2, something like anticipated regret (even though this itself is paradoxical after death!) makes us shun A_2. And in the second situation some anticipated rejoicing may induce the choice of A_3. Indulging in such feelings when making decisions is considered irrational in the context of MDA. In real life, however, anticipated regret often influences medical decisions. Heroic procedures (liver transplantation, some forms of chemotherapy) in cases of incurable cancer are a case in point. The very availability of a new and 'last resort' therapy may tempt doctors as well as patients to choose against the odds of low expected utilities.

Anticipated regret and rejoicing are instances of a principle with much wider implications in real life, viz. that preferences are often context-dependent. Values fiercely defended today may be renounced tomorrow, and this again is incompatible with the theory of MDA. Decision analysis requires that preferences are stable and transitive. If A is preferred over B and B over C, then A should be preferred over C. And such preferences should apply tomorrow, say after the operation, as well as today when we are opting for this operation. Yet in real life our behaviour often belies these assumptions. In a study of the attitudes of pregnant women towards anaesthesia during childbirth (Christensen-Szalanzki, 1984), most respondents preferred not to have anaesthesia when asked 1 month before delivery. During active labour, however, their preferences suddenly shifted towards pain avoidance by anaesthesia. When evaluating the situation 1 month after delivery, some apparently regretted this option and again expressed preference for childbirth without anaesthesia.

Context- and time-dependent preferences may of course be explained psychologically. Kahnemann and Tversky (1979) have postulated that one chooses preferences on the basis of present prospects. Thus preferences and utilities may in fact be probability-dependent. Moreover, a study by Ciampi *et al.* (1982) shows that the evaluation of a particular possible health state may depend on the actual health state of the patient. As perspectives change, so do preferences and this kind of dynamics cannot be accommodated in MDA. All this boils down to the fact that MDA theory requires a rational type of behaviour which is psychologically unrealistic. We will now take a closer look at this concept of rationality.

4. RATIONALITY AND THE ETHICS OF MDA

MDA claims to accommodate personal values and preferences. The claim, however, is conditional: provided that individuals behave rationally.

And this rational behaviour is specified: personal values should, at least in principle, be stable and transitive. MDA may even accept that, in real life, personal behaviour rarely meets this requirement and that utilities which are independent of probability or other circumstances are an idealization. MDA makes allowance for the imperfections of reality by assuming that utilities may vary within a certain range. The influence of this variability on the choice of optimal action can then be calculated (sensitivity analysis). Thus MDA's answer to irrationality is: if you must be capricious, let us at least calculate the width and weight of your caprices. MDA, and decision-analytic theory in general, guarantees efficient realization of human goals (in terms of maximum utilities), provided human behaviour adapts to at least these minimum requirements of rationality.

This strategy amounts to a reduction of human behaviour by rendering computable what is inherently unpredictable. In real life, 'other things' are never equal and the number of disturbing factors is inexhaustible. This reduction, however, is neither new nor recent. It is as old as the desire to render life's vicissitudes manageable. In western culture, this desire gained momentum in the 18th century. Engineering human happiness was a central motive in the Enlightenment and this motive was articulated in moral philosophy by, among others, Jeremy Bentham. As noted by Wulff (1976), decision-analytic theory is closely related to utilitarianism. This can be demonstrated as follows.

In *Traité de Législation* (1802), Bentham argues that the aim of a legislator should be the happiness of the people. The greatest happiness or utility is the guiding principle. On this principle, a system of reasoning is built which requires, says Bentham, that three conditions are fulfilled:

1. We must attach to the word 'utility' a clear and precise connotation.
2. We must assert the supreme and undivided sovereignty of this principle.
3. We must discover some calculus or process of 'moral arithmetic' by means of which we can arrive at uniform results.

Now if we examine the value of a pleasure or pain considered by itself and in relation to a single individual, as Bentham puts it , we shall find that it depends on four circumstances:

1. Its intensity.
2. Its duration.
3. Its certainty.
4. Its proximity.

So far Bentham.

MDA appears to be a neat elaboration of this 18th century philosophical programme. It conscientiously works out the utilitarian ideas of Jeremy Bentham. First, it attaches a clear and precise meaning to the word 'utility'. Second, MDA provides a calculus to arrive at uniform results. Furthermore, Bentham's four factors, intensity, duration, certainty and proximity, are all accounted for in MDA. One may argue that the subjective utility a person assigns to a possible outcome is based on the intensity of pleasure or pain which one thinks that this outcome may give. So intensity is dealt with in MDA. Duration is accounted for in the concept of QALYs by multiplying the value of a health state by the time spent in that state. And certainty is accounted for by MDA in that it tries to assess the probabilities of the different possible outcomes as accurately as possible. The impact of proximity in time is also dealt with in MDA. The utility function for QALYs may incorporate the idea of discounting life years in the more distant future.

It is of interest that MDA's elaboration of utilitarian principles uncovers some fundamental problems which are inherent in this type of moral reasoning. When dealing with health policy decisions, MDA renders operational 'the greatest happiness for the greatest number of citizens' by maximizing the number of QALYs (assuming cost per QALY constancy). This eliminates the problem of classical utilitarianism, viz. that the quantum of happiness and the range of distribution are separate variables to one of which decision makers will have to give priority. Using QALYs, priority is given to those groups or individuals which carry the most favourable prognosis. This, however, is in itself a specific ethical position. It may result in decisions that imply an even longer life for those who already are healthy and an even shorter life for those already diseased. In his interesting article about the non-existence of interpersonal utility scales, Hilden (1985) gives the following example: 'An upper-class woman has a longer expected life span and better health prospects throughout her life than has a lower-class woman. In a certain objective sense, she has more utility to lose in case of a premature cancer death. It would follow that it is cost-effective to spend more, relatively speaking, on cancer screening for the upper classes. This decision further reduces the expected survival of the lower-class woman. After several turns of the screw her life would simply not seem worth saving.'

But even if we renounced the criterion of maximum gain in QALYs and adhered to some kind of equal distribution of health goods over all citizens, our problems would not be over. When trying to apportion to each individual an equal chance of the same amount of utility, we assume that utility measures have interpersonal validity. In medical practice, this assumption often seems valid because doctors unwittingly apply their personal utility perceptions and patients tend to comply! However, utilities as intended in MDA are personal and cannot be averaged across individuals. Utilities, being measured on interval scales, are not anchored in an interpersonal 'reality'.

Human preferences are inherently incommensurable and Hilden therefore regards interpersonal utility scales as unrealistic. From his paper, which is here touched on only superficially, we extract the following conclusion. MDA is in fact applicable to strictly one-person decisions only, unless people accept the hypothetical commensurability of their different utility intervals.

This brings us back to the original observation that MDA requires human behaviour to conform to specific criteria of rationality. In real life, these criteria of rationality are rarely observed. Yet they are related to the utilitarian ethics of the Enlightenment and thus to the origins of modern western culture. In that period, we also find the roots of modern science and medicine and here again the concept of rationality comes into play. This concept is not a spurious postulate of MDA theory. It pervades all scientific thinking and is a central theme in philosophical analyses of modern culture. There is, however, more to it than mentioned so far.

5. FUNCTIONAL AND SUBSTANTIVE RATIONALITY

Rationality is a key concept in modern western culture, but rationality comes in different guises. Ever since Max Weber, this has been a central theme in much social philosophy. Colloquially, we implicitly assume that 'rational' and 'irrational' are unambiguous terms, known to everybody and agreed upon by all. This tacit assumption often leads to frustrations because what is self-evidently rational to A may seem incomprehensible to B. In a wider sense, 'rationality' refers to any coherent pattern or style of thought and action with which man tries to master reality. Different types of rationality characterize specific areas of human activity, types of organization, or in general, cultures and subcultures. The kind of rationality invoked by MDA is but one of these possible patterns. It is normative for much of science and for modern culture in general, but it refers to a specific style, corresponding to what Weber called 'means–ends rational action' (see Kallberg, 1980) or, in Mannheim's (1940) terminology, 'functional rationality'. Functional rationality handles reality in an instrumental way. It starts from certain objectives and focuses on ways and means for realizing these ends as effectively and efficiently as possible. Functional rationality, states Mannheim, requires that a series of actions is organized in such a way that it leads to a previously defined goal, with every element in this series of actions receiving a functional position and role. The nature of this goal is irrelevant to the rationality of this type of behaviour. One need in fact not even be cognizant of the goal or agree with it, as long as one's behaviour is organized with reference to this goal and one can adjust oneself to it in calculating one's own actions. Everything which disrupts this ordering of actions is functionally irrational. That is why MDA, as with science in general, considers the capriciousness of human behaviour as irrational. Functionally rational behaviour should be calculable in advance.

Functional rationality is a prerequisite for modern industrialized society and its scientific and technological underpinning. Without this ordering of our thoughts and actions, we could not keep the complicated machinery of our civilization running. Nor would we have developed this machinery in the first place, had not the instrumental approach to nature and to human life gained the upper hand in western culture since the 18th century. Functional rationality, however, does not help mankind in its quest, throughout history, for lasting values transcending daily routines and providing coherent meaning to the random events of life. This motive inspires what Weber called 'substantive rationality'. It strives to master reality in a value-oriented rather than in an instrumental way.

Substantive rationality directly orders actions into patterns. Unlike functional rationality, it does not do so on the basis of means–ends calculations but in relation to a 'value postulate' (see Kallberg, 1980). This implies that actors subordinate realities to values, fitting their actions into patterns which conform to specific clusters or systems of values. Examples are religious, aesthetic and moral systems which organize the behaviour of their adherents. Weber's substantive rationality implies a multitude of possible patterns of thought and action. Where values are concerned, there are no universal criteria for what is 'rational'. As our perspective changes, different configurations of values may come into view, leading to different rationalization processes. The patient who prefers a surgical intervention today and radiotherapy tomorrow may thus be perfectly rational in a value-oriented way. Regret for instance may reshuffle our preferences into a different pattern than yesterday's, but an equally 'rational' pattern.

Before applying the difference between functional and substantive rationality to our prognosis of the future of MDA, the following remarks should be made. In the first place, the scientific world view as such is a value-postulate in Weber's sense. Yet science, together with modern economics and other aspects of modernization, steered western civilization away from value-oriented action. This is demonstrated when science claims to accommodate values in its means–ends calculations. Efforts to render values measurable and calculable result in a reduction which banishes them as independent organizing principles. To Weber, this spelled the end of personal conscience and freedom. Mannheim, who used a slightly different terminology, was similarly pessimistic. The increase of functional rationality in public life forces the average man to surrender parts of his cultural individuality with every new act of integration into a functionally rationalized complex of activities (Mannheim, 1940). He becomes increasingly accustomed to being led by others and gradually gives up his own interpretation of events for those which others provide for him. How does all this apply to our evaluation of MDA?

6. CONCLUSION

As signalled in our first section, medicine is confronted with moral problems to which medical science as such has no adequate answers. MDA, when trying to provide such answers, shows itself to be a typical exponent of scientific practice and its functional rationality. In sections 2–4 we found that MDA can only pretend to deal with personal values by more or less artificial definitions or reductions of human behaviour. The solutions proffered by MDA actually circumvent the original problem. This problem, we observed in section 5, stems from the tension between functional and substantive rationality. The following examples may further clarify this tension.

Weinsten and Fineberg (1980), in their classic *Clinical Decision Analysis*, discuss the problems of utility assessment when asking for patient preferences. An individual's preferences may vary depending on the circumstances. Some people will go along with an invitation to think in terms of a risk lottery, others may be reluctant to do so. Which is the best way to approach patients? Who is the more 'valid' source of utility assessment, the patient or the physician? Throughout the argument, it is assumed that there is a 'best' or 'valid' estimate of the utility in question and the key word for this is rationality. 'Depending on the patient's mental state, rational assessments may be impossible' (Weinstein and Fineberg, 1980). As a last resort, the physician may, on the basis of documented evidence, place bounds on the preferences of the patient and decide upon the optimal strategy without making explicit estimates of the patient's unique utilities.

It is of interest that these authors admit that the optimal decision may not be the same for two patients, however similar their history, symptoms, signs and diseases may be. Utility assessments by their nature have no external validity. They do not, however, envisage the conclusion that even for a single patient there may not be one optimal decision. Functional rationality stands in the way of this conclusion. For it is postulated that medical interventions are aimed at a pre-existent goal, at an MEU, however difficult it may be to identify this goal. The idea that human goals may be moulded as they are realized, or that our life identifies its goals in retrospect, is functionally irrational. From a value-oriented perspective, however, this idea is most rational indeed. Throughout life we are searching for meaning, but we mostly find it in retrospect only. Human values are values-in-action: we define them as we live them.

Hershey and Baron (1987), in a most lucid paper on 'Clinical Reasoning and

Cognitive Processes', come close to this conclusion when they suggest that, contrary to expected utility theory, the evaluation of outcomes may be dependent on the actions that produce them. However, they do not follow up this cue beyond asking if and how decision theory should incorporate future feelings of regret. Again, functional rationality is at play. Eventual outcomes are assumed to be valued as such, i.e. as independent factual data rather than as parts of a pattern that takes shape as we live it.

Hershey and Baron's paper is most relevant to our argument because it distinguishes two major purposes of MDA: improving clinical judgment of probabilities and improving decisions. For improving clinical judgment, they think decision theory has great merit and we would like to underline this conclusion. The purpose of improving decisions, however, is more elusive. It puts MDA in a normative position which in their opinion cannot be maintained without further research about the psychological mechanisms of actual decisions in real life. However useful this recommendation may be, the problem is, in our opinion, more fundamental. MDA, like science in general, is inherently unable to improve decisions where moral problems are at stake. Our reasons for this conclusion may be summarized as follows.

As an effort to improve decisions which are traditionally intuitive or even haphazard, MDA is commendable, provided we are aware of its limitations. These limitations are related to the normativity of the theory, and of science in general, when ruling out 'irrational' behaviour. Irrationality, as we have seen, here refers to functional or means–ends rationality which is but one aspect of human life. Functional rationality may be dominant in modern culture but its very dominance is the cause of much of the moral problems with which we are confronted today. The reason is that basic human values are necessarily repressed when life is organized in a purely functional and instrumental way. In functional rationality 'values' are regarded as aspects of behaviour which can be described and analysed empirically, measured, weighed and, in brief, can be negotiated. Our need for substantive rationality, on the other hand, invokes values in a different way. Here values direct our behaviour as organizing principles which can only be described evocatively. They can be adhered to or renounced, but not calculated. Most importantly, they become manifest biographically as we review our past and present.

It should be noted that both connotations of 'values' may exist side by side and the one may shade off into the other. Friendship, for example, may mean liking someone and wanting to be in his or her company. As such it may well be weighed and negotiated. In another sense, however, friendship has a connotation of loyalty, of 'right or wrong, my friend', and as such may lead us to functionally irrational behaviour. Quality is another example and may serve to conclude our argument. Quality may be the sum of a number of positive attributes or faculties. Thus a Karnofsky index may measure quality of life. This is quality as an extra to quantity, quality of life as an extra to survival. Measurable and negotiable, this quality is a value as conceived by MDA. In substantive rationality, on the other hand, quality may appear in many shapes but it is always an absolute, an essence, which cannot be described analytically. Such quality is fundamental to the phenomena it characterizes (Pirsig, 1976; 'Real quality must be the source of the subjects and objects') and cannot be isolated as an 'extra'. When quality is experienced as the essence of life, the very word 'life' takes on a different meaning and the idea of life as mere duration becomes a contradiction in terms.

We started from the observation that modern medicine is in trouble because of the tensions between medical science on the one hand and the realities of medical practice on the other. These problems are most acute at the frontiers of medicine's successful expansion. Ethical problems in advanced oncology, neonatology and intensive care in general are cases in point. The expansion of modern medicine at the expense of primary care, leading to social injustices, is another example. In all of these, we may see functional rationality over-reaching its range of control. MDA cannot change such problems since it is part and parcel of this same rationality. It may follow medicine as a useful addition to its methodology but it can never be a remedy for medicine's shortcomings. In these frontier areas, man has to fall back on prescientific substantive rationality, which means that ultimately, when confronted with decisions which affect the meaning of our personal and social life, we have to renounce the rationality of science and medicine. The surfeit of medical success calls for a restoration of balance and an awareness of the limits of scientific control. The coming moral crisis of medicine can be overcome only if we revive a sense of the most basic fact and value of life: its finiteness.

REFERENCES

Bentham, J. (1802) *Traité de Législation Civile et Pénale*, vol. I. Bossange, Masson et Besson, Paris, (for translation purposes we consulted C.M.A. Atkinson's English version, *Theory of Legislation*, Clarendon Press, Oxford, 1914) pp. 1, 51.

Christensen-Szalanski, J. J. J. (1984) Discount functions and the measurement of patients' values. Women's decisions during childbirth. *Medical Decision Making* **4**, 47–58.

Ciampi, A., Silberfeld, M. and Till, J. E. (1982) Measurement of individual preferences. The importance of situation-specific variables. *Medical Decision Making* **4**, 483–95.

Hershey, J. C. and Baron, J. B. (1987) Clinical reasoning and cognitive processes. *Medical Decision Making* **7**, 203–11.

Hilden J. (1985) The nonexistence of interpersonal utility scales. *Medical Decision Making* **5**, 215–28.

Kahnemann, D. and Tversky, A. (1979) Prospect theory: an analysis of decision under risk. *Econometrica* **47**, 263–91.

Kallberg, S. (1980) Max Weber's types of rationality: cornerstones for the analysis of rationalization processes in history. *American Journal of Sociology* **85**, 1145–79.

Mannheim, K. (1940) *Man and Society in an Age of Reconstruction*. Kegan Paul, Trench and Trubner, London, pp. 53–9.

McNeil, B. J., Weichselbaum, R. and Pauker, S. G. (1981) Speech and survival; tradeoffs between quality and quantity of life on laryngeal cancer. *New England Journal of Medicine* **305**, 982–7.

Mooney, G. (1989) Qaly's: are they enough? *Journal of Medical Ethics* (in press).

Najman, J. M. and Levine, S. (1981) Evaluating the impact of medical care and technologies on the quality of life. *Social Science and Medicine* **15F**, 107–15.

Pirsig, R. M. (1976) *Zen and the Art of Motorcycle Maintenance*. Corgi Books, London, p. 286.

Pliskin, J. S. and Pliskin, N. (1980) Decision analysis in clinical practice. *European Journal of Operational Research* **4**, 153–9.

Pliskin, J. S., Shepard, D. S. and Weinstein, M. C. (1980) Utility functions for life years and health status. *Operations Research* **28**, 206–24.

Sugden, R. (1985) Regret, recrimination and rationality. *Theory and Decision* **19**, 77–99.

Sutherland, H. J., Llewellyn-Thomas, H., Boyd, N. F. and Till, J. E. (1982) Attitudes toward quality of survival; the concept of 'maximal endurable time'. *Medical Decision Making* **2**, 299–309.

van der Steen, W. J. and Thung, P. J. (1988) *Faces of Medicine, A Philosophical Study*. Reidel, Dordrecht, Chapter II.

Von Neumann, J. and Morgenstern, O. (1944) *Theory of Games and Economic Behavior*. Princeton University Press, Princeton.

Warndorff, D. K., Pouls, C. J. M. and Knottnerus, J. A. (1988) Medische besliskunde in Nederland. *Medisch Contact* **43**, 1174–8.

Weinstein, M. C. and Fineberg, H. V. (1980) *Clinical Decision Analysis*. Saunders, Philadelphia, pp. 220–2.

Wulff, H. R. (1976) *Rational Diagnosis and Treatment*. Blackwell, Oxford.

7

Social Change and the Perception of Risks in Medical Practice

Roel Otten, Drs and Guy Widdershoven, PhD

1. INTRODUCTION

Medical practice involves risks for patients. These risks are, however, perceived differently by the different persons involved. It is well known that a layman's view of risks in technical enterprises is not the same as the view of an expert. Similarly the view of the patient will diverge from that of the medical practitioner. It is often thought that these differences can be explained by cognitive factors. Experts know the objective risks, whereas the general public is easily influenced by emotional feelings of fear and panic. This cognitive approach to risk perception presupposes that risks can be objectively measured and that changes in risk perception are related to growth of objective knowledge. The expert's judgment of a risk is seen as more valuable than the perception of a layman, because the first is based on objective knowledge of the world. Against this it may be argued, however, that there exists no such thing as an objective, value-free risk. Even a specialist's perception of risks is biased. An estimation of risks is someone's estimation. Statistical analysis for instance does not only imply the accumulation of information, transferred in mathematical models by a computer. The information used is selected information and a belief in the exactness of the analysis is based on a judgment on the relevance of this information (Rayner, 1984, 1986).

In this chapter we will argue that differences and changes in risk perception are not a purely cognitive matter. What people see as a risk depends on values which are highly influenced by social factors. Selection of information and thus the perception of risks always presupposes values on basis of which

Changing Values in Medical and Health Care Decision Making
Edited by U. J. Jensen and G. Mooney

one selects. According to Mary Douglas these values are cultural constructs which are deeply rooted in one's place in a social environment. This is further explicated in her so-called group–grid theory which aims at analysing the structure of a social environment and the associated values and attitudes towards risks (Douglas, 1970, 1978; Douglas and Wildavsky, 1982).

We will concentrate here on differences in values and risk perception between general practitioners and specialists. First we will present two medical malpractice trials. By comparing the way in which the specialist and the general practitioner defend themselves in these trials, we will make clear that there are differences in their value systems and consequently in their perception of risks in medical treatments. Next we will explain these differences by making use of Mary Douglas's group–grid analysis, in which social structures are related to value systems (or cosmologies). The value system of specialists is such that they tend to pay most attention to short-term risks. General practitioners are more open to long-term risks, such as the risk of medicalization. These differences can be explained by differences in the structure of their social environment.

Social structure also influences the perception of the way in which risks can be dealt with. Specialists tend to define their practice as instrumental, whereas general practitioners have a more complex view of medical practice. Given the relationship between social structure, value systems and risk perception we will conclude that not only growth of knowledge, but also changes in the social structure of general practitioners and specialists may lead to changes in their values and consequently in the way they perceive risks and deal with these risks.

2. TWO MEDICAL MALPRACTICE TRIALS

On 19 January 1981 a complaint against a general practitioner was brought before a Dutch medical disciplinary committee. The general practitioner was accused by a former patient of not having treated her breast complaint adequately. After a not totally unambiguous mammography the doctor had said there was nothing wrong, without sending the patient to a specialist. Later it appeared that her complaints were caused by breast cancer. The general practitioner defended himself by saying that 90% of all non-palpable tumours are localized by a mammography and that the woman did not belong to a high-risk group. He also mentioned that patients should be protected against unnecessary fear of cancer. The disciplinary committee convicted the practitioner and pronounced that each woman undergoing a mammography should be investigated by a specialist, who knows exactly how to palpate the breast.

The case did not go unnoticed. An unusually large number of letters about it were published in the Dutch medical journal *Medisch Contact*. Several general practitioners disagreed with the judgment. They claimed that specialists do not always know best. General practitioners, so it was said, have their own responsibilities, which include guarding against the dangers of somatic fixation and cancer phobia. In view of this more general task, the risks involved in not sending a patient to a specialist might be acceptable. It was said that for a general practitioner, although mammography might not be optimal, it was still the most useful diagnostic instrument. Most of the general practitioners felt that the disciplinary committee was to blame, not the doctor, because its judgment denied any meaning for the work of the general practitioner.

On 28 January 1969 an anaesthetist was charged in the law courts in Amsterdam by an inspector of public health. In spite of several complications with a narcosis during a relatively simple operation, the anaesthetist had agreed to continue. After the operation the patient appeared to be decerebrated. The anaesthetist was accused of not having judged the situation adequately. According to the inspector he should have postponed the operation, since it was not an urgent one. Several experts were heard in court. Their opinion on the seriousness of the situation was rather divergent. As to the acceptability of the risk, most anaesthetists questioned in court supported the accused. It was said that in 9 out of 10 cases an anaesthetist would be able to manage a similar problem. The anaesthetist was acquitted.

Although the cases described above are not exactly comparable, the contrast between the two is evident. In the case of the general practitioner, a risk of 10% was judged by the medical disciplinary committee as unacceptable. For the anaesthetist a 10% risk was said to be acceptable, both by his colleagues and by the court of law. In the first case the disciplinary committee thought the risk was too high because the somatic factor, which is regarded as the most important one, was not adequately dealt with. The patient should have been investigated by a specialist. The general practitioners questioned the assumption that only the somatic aspects are relevant. Besides physiological abnormalities, they wanted to pay attention to fear of cancer and somatic fixation. In the second case both the court and the experts saw the risks as acceptable provided all somatic factors were thoroughly investigated and interpreted correctly. General practitioners and specialists differed in their opinion as to which factors were relevant and how these factors should be dealt with. The authorities tended to agree with the specialists' point of view rather than with that of the general practitioners.

3. GROUP AND GRID

Douglas defines the structure of a social group by two dimensions: group and grid. The group dimension is a measure of the extent to which individuals in their interaction with others are constrained by their membership of a group. 'High group' stands for groups with a strong emphasis on a group boundary, resulting in a division of the world between 'us' and 'the others'. This is in contrast with 'low group' where there is not so much emphasis on the division between us and the others. 'Grid' says something about the extent to which persons are constrained in their relationships with others by role differentiation. 'High grid' implies the existence of a highly differentiated and hierarchical role system. Grid is 'low' when access to different roles is not based on a given order but depends on negotiation or conventions. If both dimensions are related to each other there are four different social structures. To each of these social structures belongs a particular value system. This value system determines the way in which people perceive risks. We will describe these four different types of social structure together with their typical value system and the way in which this influences the perception of risks, using risks in nuclear industry as an example (Gross and Rayner, 1985).

3.1. High group–high grid

In this social context the driving force behind peoples' actions is the maintenance of the system as a whole in which each individual has a specific role. The bureaucratic organization is a good example. The emphasis is laid on correctly applying existing formal procedures or rules—the ritual. The attitude of the bureaucrat against the dangers of nuclear power will be influenced by his strong belief in formal procedures and rules which will alarm the organization in time. People in this environment will not be afraid of technological dangers because there are procedures to deal with them. The real danger in this context is the loss of confidence in the organization.

3.2. Low group–low grid

Because of the absence of an explicit group boundary and the absence of a strong natural given role differentiation, this social context has optimal opportunities for the individual. Prestige and influence are in principle attainable for everyone. But on the other hand everybody is responsible for his own actions. This social context is best compared with a free market situation. Everybody strives to maximize his own position. The behaviour that best pays off in this situation is not to ignore or regret uncertainty. On the contrary, risks are opportunities. In relation to ideas about nuclear power, this cosmology leads to the opinion that no technological advance that brought the pleasures of modern time was or is without risks. A second aspect that contributes to the low group–low grid perception of the dangers of nuclear power is a short-term view of risks. Low group–low grid people will not be very sensitive to the argument that nuclear waste will be a danger for future generations. On the contrary, they will lay emphasis on the fact that new technologies will cope with this problem.

3.3. Low group–high grid

This environment can be characterized by a refined, strong hierarchical structure, without a clear group process which supports this structure. In this social context the largest group of people has no control over other people, goods or capital and no access to the main centres of control. For their access to goods, capital etc. they are dependent on people who take a more central place in the social network. People in this context cannot manipulate but are constantly being manipulated by others. That is why they distrust experts. They will demonstrate against the dangers of nuclear power on the basis of a concrete fear of disturbance of their live-world. A second aspect in their attitude to nuclear power is that they feel that they have to bear the risks in favour of the people who have the power. Because time develops constantly and regularly in this context, they feel threatened by slow developing dangers like leakage of radiation and give less attention to short-term risks like, for instance, a meltdown.

3.4. High group–low grid

This environment lays strong emphasis on the group boundary. With regard to the grid dimension, all aspects of social relationships are open to negotiations and conventions. Decisions are being taken on the basis of consensus. Solidarity is the most important value. Because of this emphasis on solidarity and brotherhood it is to be expected that groups with such a structure will see bureaucratic and free-market groups as threatening and even as evil. They will see events that go with these groups as extremely risky. Nuclear power is a capital-intensive energy source that can only be controlled by large organizations with a central, hierarchical centre of control. Because of this, nuclear power is seen as a great risk by high group–low grid groups.

4. THE SOCIAL ENVIRONMENT OF GENERAL PRACTITIONERS AND SPECIALISTS

Having outlined the theoretical framework within which we can analyse the way people select risks, we turn back to the malpractice trials of the general practitioner and the anaesthetist. First we will describe the social environment of these two in terms of group and grid. Next, we will show

GRID		
high	**B** Residual Constrained by rules Obligations and demands imposed by classification but few resources from others Fragmented networks Risks imposed by others without consultation – passive resentment Future seen as endless repetition of operational cycles	**C** Bureaucratic Hierarchical Constrained by rules but also protected by them Many demands and resources derived from others Highly structured networks with distinct boundaries Risks routinized through established procedures – complacency Expectations of future based on past epochs marked by ancestors or great events
low	**A** Competitive Market Unconstrained by rules Few demands or resources from others Ego-centred networks without boundaries Risks incorporated into portfolios of concerns – acceptance of calculated risks Future incorporated in concern for operational deadlines	**D** Egalitarian Group Unconstrained by rules Many demands and resources from others Transitive networks with distinct boundaries Risks resisted – high sensitivity to possible hazards Future epochs compressed into the present on model of short historical depth
0	low	high GROUP

Grid and group dimensions and associated attitudes to risk and the future

that the value system belonging to their social structure is identifiable in the way they defended themselves in the medical malpractice trials earlier described.

Eliot Freidson's analysis of the situation of the general practitioner gives some clues to describe the group–grid structure of the general practitioner (Freidson, 1970). He concludes that the general practitioner's practice is mainly patient-centred. The decision to go and see a general practitioner is based on a lay opinion. As shown in the case of the general practitioner, the problems of a patient consist of a mixture of social, psychological and medical factors. If a general practitioner wants to keep his patients—and thus his practice—in the future, he has to meet the needs of his patients in such way that they feel helped. Of course, besides the demands of his patients, the general practitioner also has to meet medical standards. The ultimate medical standard is set by committees like the medical disciplinary committee. But according to the general practitioners, these committees are basically focused on the situation of specialists, using norms which are consistent with specialists' norms. Based on these two insights we describe the environment of the general practitioner as high grid. He is part of a social network in which he has no possibility to manipulate others, but on the contrary is being manipulated by patients and medical disciplinary committees.

To say something about the group dimension, it is important to establish if the general practitioner acts in his own interest or in the interest of a group. Although there do exist different types of co-operations on different levels in which general practitioners work together, the general practitioner is basically an entrepreneur in competition with others. His practice has to have a minimal size to be commercially profitable. Besides, the general practitioner does not spend much of his time with others. He works basically alone. Based on these two criteria, we characterize the social environment of the general practitioner as low group. So we conclude that the general practitioner works in a low group–high grid context.

We now turn to the social environment of the specialist. At first sight this seems to exhibit a high group–high grid structure. There is a marked division of labour in which everybody has a narrow, delineated task. These roles are not accessible to everybody, not even for all people within the group of specialists. The training in a particular specialty takes years and after that it is not possible to take up a totally different specialty. The anaesthetist for instance cannot become an orthopaedist from one day to the next. Moreover, specialists are totally dependent on each other during an operation. Without the assistance of an anaesthetist it would be impossible for the heart surgeon to operate. However, we do not think that the environment of the anaesthetist should be described as high group–high grid. Again, Freidson offers some clues (Freidson, 1970). He describes in detail the mechanisms that specialists use to control other colleagues. There are no formal procedures to keep one another in line, only informal ones. The only real controlling activity specialists use is best described as 'let's talk'. This means that if a specialist is out of line one of his colleagues will try to get him back in line through an informal chat. If this fails to work a second mechanism comes into play, which is best described as 'keeping the nest clean'. People make sure they are no longer associated with the colleague who has a bad name. We conclude that the social environment of the specialist should not be described as high group–high grid, but as low group–low grid. There is no formal structure which rules the relationships between specialists. Prosperity and misfortune are not affairs of collective but of personal responsibility. As soon as the personal position of specialists is endangered, everybody draws his own conclusions at an individual level. They work together because they need each other and they will support each other, for instance in malpractice trials, but only to the extent that there is no danger to their personal status. At this point group behaviour changes to egocentric behaviour.

5. THE VALUE SYSTEMS OF GENERAL PRACTITIONER AND SPECIALIST

The social structure in which the general practitioner is situated can, we argued, be characterized in terms of low group and high grid. The value system of the low group–high grid category has two aspects. In the first place representatives of this category resist disturbances in their life situation, especially those disturbances caused by people who are more central in the network. In the second place they tend to emphasize the long-term consequences of decisions. The first aspect is easily recognized in the reactions of the general practitioners against the verdict of the medical disciplinary committee. The general practitioners make a stand against the excessive influence of specialists on the committee. They argue that specialists are not able to judge the situation of a general practitioner. The committee is blamed for its undermining of the position of general practitioners.

The emphasis on long-term consequences is also prominent in the reactions of the general practitioners. The accused general practitioner mentions fear of cancer, a factor which in the long run might harm the patient. The notions of 'somatic fixation' and 'cancer phobia', used by other general practitioners, refer to comparable long-term consequences. A central argument against rashly sending a patient to a specialist is the menace of medicalization. This is a long-term undesirable consequence of apparently harmless individual decisions. The extent to which general practitioners are receptive to the problem of medicalization fits very well in the low group–high grid value system.

In the discussion on the social structure of the specialist we argued for a low group–low grid classification. In contrast to the low group–high grid category, this category is not conservative, but opportunistic and pragmatic. Emphasis is not laid on resistance against interference of others but on the justification of risks by current experts. A second aspect of the low group–low grid value system is a short-term perspective on the future. Both aspects can be found in the specialists' perception of risks. Specialists underline the need for expert judgment. In defending his decision, the accused anaesthetist stressed that he himself was the expert, qualified to judge the situation. This claim was supported by another anaesthetist heard in court. The specialists tend to see only short-term consequences. The accused specialist and the other specialists who were questioned only spoke about directly controllable factors. As long as these factors are all considered, the decision is seen as acceptable.

Social structure and the related value system not only influence the perception of risks, but also the perception of the way in which risks can be dealt with. Ostrander (1982) argues that people in the low group–low grid category regard the separation of nature and society as progress. Man conquers nature through his own ingenuity and for his own benefit. This implies a positive outlook on the possibilities of instrumental action. In the low group–high grid category the social order is seen as a constant danger which cannot be manipulated easily. The situation in which one has to act is seen as complex. Instrumental action alone is in this perspective insufficient to solve the main problems with which people have to deal.

These different views on human action can be recognized in the two cases we discussed above. The specialists stress the importance of adequate instrumental action. The general practitioners have a more complex view of the situation and their own practice. According to the specialists medical practice is technical. According to the general practitioner it is something more, and different.

6. CHANGE IN SOCIAL STRUCTURE, VALUE SYSTEM AND RISK PERCEPTION

One feature of Mary Douglas's group–grid theory is its explicit static typology. It simply says that each of the four social contexts is related to a particular kind of value system. According to Douglas, social structure and value system are two aspects of one system which keep each other in balance so that they constitute a dynamic but stable equilibrium. Her theory aims to explain social stability but cannot be used to explain social instability or social change and possible changes in risk perception as a result of this social change.

In his interpretation of the group–grid theory, Michael Thompson introduces a third variable, which together with the variables group and grid can account for social instability or social change (Thompson, 1982a,b). According to Thompson, people in a given group–grid configuration can only use certain strategies to improve their situation. This third variable, which Thompson calls 'manipulation', is a measure of the extent to which people in a given social context are in a position to manipulate others. Without specifying what this means for individuals in all four group–grid configurations, we will describe which type of manipulation pays off for individuals in a high grid–low group environment. People in this environment find themselves at the periphery of a social network and are therefore easy to manipulate. Their only chance to improve their situation lies in decreasing the grid component of their context, at least for them. The only way to achieve this is to build their own social network in which they themselves take a more central place. In other words, they will be moving to a social context with low group and low grid.

The reactions of the general practitioners to the verdict of the medical disciplinary committee can, in our opinion, be understood in this way. The practitioners hold that they no longer want to be judged by these kind of medical disciplinary committees simply because these committees do not know the problems with which they have to deal. According to the general practitioners it is time that they had their own system of evaluation. In this way it becomes possible for the general practitioners to build their own social network in which they can play a more central role with their own specialty and evaluation of this specialty. The general practitioners' plea for their own disciplinary committee, served only by general practitioners, can be seen as a way to strive to a more central place in a social network. If this should succeed, their social structure would change from high grid–low group to low grid–low group. Consequently their value system would change, which at the same time would result in a change of their perception of risks in medical treatments. They would lay more emphasis on individual expertise and on an opportunistic attitude towards risks. If Thompson's extension of the group–grid theory has some strength, and we believe it has, it accounts for possible changes in risk perception among general practitioners not in terms of growth of knowledge but in terms of changes in their value system, connected with changes in the structure of their social environment.

7. CONCLUSIONS

In this chapter we have argued that the sociological group–grid theory can account for the values that play a role in the perception of risks by the general practitioners and specialists. The value system of the general practitioner is such that he is sensitive to the interference of others—specialists and patients—and tends to emphasize long-term risks against which instrumental action alone is not sufficient. In contrast with the general practitioner, the specialist emphasizes the short-term consequences of risks and stresses the importance of expert judgment and the importance of instrumental action in situations with which he has to deal. Social structure and value system however, are not totally static. People in the periphery of a social network, such as general practitioners, strive for a more central place in the network. If they succeed, their value system and thus the way they perceive risks in medical treatments will change as well.

Although the group–grid theory fits well with the different lines of defence chosen by the general practitioners and the specialists, there are also other possible explanations for the differences in risk perception in the cases described. One may notice that specialists and general practitioners have different populations of patients, which ask for a different approach. General practitioners, it may be said, have a far more diverse population than specialists whose population of patients is much easier to define. Although epidemiological factors are surely relevant, it is our conviction that they are not solely responsible for the difference in risk perception between specialists and general practitioners. In support of a sociological analysis, it may be noted that specialists who have a less central position in the medical network have a cosmology which shows strong resemblance to the cosmology of general practitioners.

An analysis of the differences between various types of specialists might be the next step in judging the merits of a sociological analysis of differences in risk perception. We believe the group–grid theory to be a useful instrument, not only in explaining why people select risks in the way they do, but also in making us sensitive to possible risk scenarios we might expect as a result of changes in organization in certain parts of health care systems or health care systems as a whole.

REFERENCES

Douglas, M. (1970) *Natural Symbols*. Barrie & Rockliffe, London.

Douglas, M. (1978) *Cultural Bias*. Royal Anthropological Institute Occasional Paper No. 35, London.

Douglas, M. and Wildavsky, A. (1982) *Risk and Culture*. University of California Press, Berkeley.

Freidson, E. (1970) *Profession of Medicine: A Study of the Sociology of Applied Knowledge*. Harper & Row, New York.

Gross, J. L. and Rayner, S. (1985) *Measuring Culture: A Paradigm for the Analysis of Social Organization*. Columbia University Press, New York.

Ostrander, D. (1982) One- and two-dimensional models of the distribution of beliefs. In: Douglas, M. (ed.) *Essays in the Sociology of Perception*. Routledge & Kegan Paul, London, pp. 14–30.

Rayner, S. (1984) Disagreeing about risks: the institutional cultures of risk management and planning for future generations. In: Hadden, S. (ed.) *Risk Analysis, Institutions and Public Policy*. Associated Faculty Press, Port Washington, pp. 150–69.

Rayner, S. (1986) Management of radiation hazards in hospitals: plural rationalities in a single institution. *Social Studies of Science* **16**, 537–91.

Thompson, M. (1982a) A three-dimensional model. In: Douglas, M. (ed.) *Essays in the Sociology of Perception*. Routledge & Kegan Paul, London, pp. 31–63.

Thompson, M. (1982b) The problem of the centre: an autonomous cosmology. In: Douglas, M. (ed.) *Essays in the Sociology of Perception*. Routledge & Kegan Paul, London, pp. 302–27.

8

Health Care Need, Values and Change: How Changed Values Influence an Evaluative Concept

Per-Erik Liss, BA and Lennart Nordenfelt, PhD

1. INTRODUCTION

It is not certain that a good society would be a society in which we all got what we wanted. That society, however, does not exist and probably never will, because although there are natural limits on resources, there seem to be no natural limits on our preferences. We have to constrain these preferences, and not just for ethical reasons. It is important that the restriction is not arbitrary, especially when we shape our institutions. How, for instance, health care is allocated affects us in several important respects.

However, here we shall not devote our time to the question as to what, if any, criteria it would be possible or rational to choose for the purpose of allocation—a choice in which values would certainly be involved. What we intend rather is to consider a criterion or concept which is often suggested and examine to what extent or in what respect it contains values and thereby is susceptible to changes in values. The idea of *need* pervades social services and it also pervades the social policies that shape the institutions under whose aegis those services are conducted. For instance, the Swedish Public Health Act lays down that the policies of the health care system should be determined only by the needs of patients.

It is also legitimate to ask how changeable people's health care needs are. It might be different to use health care needs as a foundation for planning or priority setting if they change too readily or quickly. Planning health services in accordance with need means taking future needs into consideration.

Changing Values in Medical and Health Care Decision Making
Edited by U. J. Jensen and G. Mooney

People's basic needs seem not to have changed much over time. The reason might be quite simple. Basic human needs are tied to human nature and the nature of the creature called *Homo sapiens* has hardly changed at all. Health care need, on the other hand, is not tied to human nature in the same sense and is therefore more susceptible to change.

Health care needs are mostly influenced by diseases. A variation in diseases is likely to lead to a variation in the need for health care. Diseases may be influenced or caused, in their turn, by a number of different factors, such as climate, social structure, material standard of living of the culture, means of production, lifestyle, etc. Changes in values certainly influence changes in at least some of these factors. For instance, choice of lifestyle is a choice based on values. Today we know what effect lifestyle may have on disease patterns. Changes in values may in this way lead to changes in people's need for health care.

There is, however, another issue here which is important with regard to this chapter. When we assess the need for care of a specific individual, or of a whole population, we normally use some kind of standard or criterion of what should count as a health care need. This criterion is based on a view of what a need for health care is. When we change this concept, we also change the need for health care. Thus, it is possible that a population's need for health care is changed not by, for instance, a change in the disease pattern, but by a change in the concept of health care need.

If we so wished, we could dramatically cut down the scope of a population's need for health care by using a certain concept of need, a concept which perhaps mirrors our low ambitions concerning health. But we could also do just the opposite. We could be ambitious and define the concept in a generous way, which would result in an increased health care need in the population.

Now, at this point certain urgent questions might make themselves heard. Is it possible to *choose* the features of health care need, or do we have to discover them? (We have so far assumed the former.) Is the concept of health care need a value-laden concept which is susceptible to changes in values? If so, in what ways is it value-laden? What components in the concept of health care need are susceptible to changes in values?

In the following sections we shall try to answer these questions. We will then argue that the concept of need contains components which we cannot discover but have to choose, and that health care need therefore might change when values change. We will specify those components and discuss what factors might have an influence on them. Finally, we will deal with the intricate question of whose values should have a determining influence on the definition of health care need—and thus have a determining effect on people's need for health care. We shall start by presenting some of the basic features of the concept of health care need.

2. THE CONCEPT OF HEALTH CARE NEED

The concepts of need and health care need, despite their importance in different circumstances, remain confused and sometimes confusing, all the more so because the confusion frequently passes unacknowledged. The confusion is partly due to the multi-faceted natures of the concepts. We refer to at least *three different things* with the term 'need'. First, it can be and has been connected with *motives or drives*. A living organism strives to keep itself in balance. It is said to be struggling to maintain homeostasis. Disturbances, induced by internal or external stimuli, lead to tensions in the organism. Sometimes the term 'need' is used to designate these tensions. (The concept of a tension-need is defined in Liss, 1986.)

We can agree about the possibility of, for instance, a tension-need for water or alcohol (in some form), but there is unlikely to exist a tension-need for health care. This type of need is therefore not of interest in this context.

Assume now a situation where we say that Mr Smith has a need for care. This locution is typically used when Smith lacks care, when he has not yet obtained care. In such a locution the term 'need' refers to *a state of lack* or, as we have argued elsewhere, *a difference* between what is and what ought to be (Liss, 1986).

It is common to use the term 'need' in a third way. We can say that care is a need of Smith's, or that food or love is a human need. The term 'need' here refers to what we need, to what shall be called *the object of need*.

It is important to notice the difference between the object of need and the need (as a difference). There seem to be no restrictions on what things we can need (except impossible things), and any overlooking of the distinction between need and the object of need might lead to confusion and to the view that need is something very complex and simply indefinable.

Beyond these initial clarifications, let us try to understand the concept of need. What is it somebody has, more exactly, when he or she has a need for something? We shall start by considering the logical structure of the concept.

When we have a need, we do not only have a need *for* something—we also need this something in order to reach or obtain some goal. We, for instance, need food in order to live, love in order to live well, health care in order to stay or become healthy, and so on. We can illustrate this idea in the following way: 'P has a need for X in order to Y'. What P needs X in order to—Y in this case—will be called *the goal of need*, and what P needs or has a need for—X in this case—is *the object of need*.

The important function of the goal of need should be noticed. It determines what things (X) we need. For a given P, a change in Y leads to a change in X. We need, for instance, other things for a holiday on a summer beach than for a holiday in the snow. Or in other words, what we need varies with, for instance, how we plan to spend our life. We need other things if we want to live as a farmer than if we want to manage a hospital in the city. Some needs are, of course, common to most life-plans, because they probably involve such common goals as 'survival' or 'decent standard of living'. But as the total sets of goals vary as well as the means of reaching the goals, the subjects' total lists of what they need will have different contents.

Now, with respect to health care need, the goals of need will determine the quantity and quality of the care needed. To try to decide what we need could only be a form of speculation as long as we do not have a clear picture of the goal of need. Here we could rightly speak of an instrumental view of need. The satisfaction of a need is instrumental for some goal.

The concept of need could be defined in the following way.

> P has a need of X in situation S if, and only if, (1) there is a difference in S between an actual state of P and a goal G, and (2) X is in S a necessary condition for G.

We can see that if condition (1) is fulfilled there is a need, and if both (1) and (2) are fulfilled there is a need of X. If we substitute health care for X we have a definition of health care need.

We can understand from this analysis of need that a need is met when the gap is eliminated. And we can eliminate the gap either by manipulating the actual state or by changing the goal, or both. What we first think of is, of course, to manipulate the actual state, that is, to give care or cure. But in principle it is possible to eliminate a need by lowering our ambitions. The goal could be lowered from, for instance, 'fit for work' to 'get on by himself at home'. We would say that we *meet* a need when we manipulate the actual state, but we *eliminate* a need when we change the goal.

3. HEALTH CARE NEED AND VALUE

Where there are values involved there are often disagreements. Let us therefore briefly examine in what way disagreements about need could arise. Suppose there are disagreements about the use of a certain medical treatment. Such a disagreement could originate in at least three different factors. First, it could be a disagreement about the person's actual state: in what bodily or mental condition is the person? Perhaps the person does not need extra vitamins (as he or she thinks) because it is not required by his or her condition (according to the doctor). Second, disagreement could arise about *the goal of need*, about that state of affairs which it is desirable to reach with the care or the treatment. Perhaps it would be satisfactory even if he or she did not reach complete health, or perhaps this would be quite unsatisfactory.

Notice that there is a difference here between these disagreements. The first was about an actual state of a person, about facts regarding the person's condition. This condition may be described in different terms, for example in terms of health or lack of health. The second disagreement was about a goal: what state of affairs it would be desirable to reach with the care or the treatment. Generally speaking, facts are discovered but goals are chosen, and the latter involve values in a way the former do not.

Third, even if the doctor and the patient after all agree on both the actual state and the goal, they can still disagree about the need of a certain treatment. The patient might not accept the secondary effects of the suggested treatment or the doctor might think the requested treatment not worthwhile. We have here a disagreement about the object of need, about a suitable treatment or means of reaching the goal of need. Sometimes there is only one treatment available, but in many cases we have a choice, including the possibility of renouncing treatment altogether.

We can conclude from this brief examination that values are involved in health care need in at least two ways. Both the goal of need and the suitable treatment to reach the goal are things we *choose*.

What kind of treatment ought to be chosen in a certain case is of course nothing we can or should deal with here. It would not be out of place, however, to say something about the goal of need. We could always discuss what goal it would be reasonable to choose when assessing the need for health care of an individual patient or of an entire population. It would be possible, for instance, to base a choice of the goal on an outlook on life or some kind of theory of value or theory of justice (an example of the latter is presented in Daniels, 1985). But it is also possible to take a more pragmatic position and let the purpose of providing health care have a determining effect on the choice of goal. Preserved or improved *health* is probably a goal which is common to every health care system.

3.1. Theories of health

In what ways, if any, are values involved in the concept of health? A first answer is perhaps not unexpected: it depends on how we look upon health. Two very different types of theories of health can be found in the theoretical discourse on medicine: an analytical and a holistic type.

In the *analytical* type statistical normality is the key concept. Man is claimed to have certain normal characteristics concerning both structure and function. We can observe how these characteristics contribute to the survival of the individual or to the survival of the species. A species-typical design appears. Scientists can detect the species-typical design of man by inspecting a large sample of human beings, by making a biostatistical analysis. For instance, the species-typical pulse rate of man consists of that interval range in which most people's pulses can be found.

An analytical theory of health is presented in Boorse (1977). The theory is analysed and commented on in Nordenfelt (1987). The basic idea in the analytical theory is that diseases are internal states which interfere with the normal functioning of the organism. There is a disease if, and only if, the function of an organ deviates in a subnormal way from the species-typical function. The whole person is ill, according to the theory, when he or she has an organ which functions subnormally. Health is then defined in terms of disease: a person is healthy if, and only if, he or she has no disease. No attention is in this theory paid to the performance of the organism in a larger, for instance social, context.

The analysis of this theory in Nordenfelt (1987) pays much attention to the concept of a function, and the relation between an organism's functional ability and its environment. Two major points are made in the analysis.

1. The analytical theory is not a clear theory of health or disease unless we know at what level of integration the biological functions are to be identified. We get very different results if the relevant functions are interpreted to be, on the one hand, the functions of the microscopic parts of the body, or, on the other hand, the gross functions of the major organs. Both of these extreme alternatives can yield counter-intuitive consequences.
2. The theory faces a number of difficulties when we consider more closely the dynamic interaction between an organism and the environmental change pertaining to the organism. The latter point may be illustrated by an example of an ordinary infection (Nordenfelt, 1987).

In a paradigm case of an infection a number of microbes invade a tissue. They start producing toxins and destroy a number of cells. The body reacts and starts to defend itself against the attack: blood concentrates at the focal point of the infection; antibodies are created; the body temperature rises, etc. This defence is a species-typical reaction to an attack on the body, and is therefore not a disease, according to the analytical theory. Paradoxically, then, a typical disease is seen, given the analytical theory, as a healthy response to a difficult environment.

In ordinary medical discourse infections are viewed as diseases. The reason for this must then be something other than considerations concerning statistical normality. We find the most probable reason to be that infections normally affect the whole person—for instance, his or her ability to function in a social context.

The analysis of the analytical theory shows that it has serious defects and that it cannot adequately reflect the concept of health either in ordinary discourse or in medical practice (Nordenfelt, 1987). This conclusion provides good reason for considering a theory where pain and disability play an essential role—a theory constructed from a holistic perspective.

The *holistic* theories focus on the human being as a whole. According to them the function and activity of the entire person is conclusive for our judgment of a person's health. Particulars are important only as causal factors behind the functioning of the whole. An everyday formulation of this holistic idea is that a person is healthy if he or she feels well and can function in his or her social context. Here health is the more basic concept and disease is defined in terms of health. Diseases are characterized as such bodily and mental states or processes as tend to compromise health.

The basic idea in the holistic theory, put forward by Nordenfelt, is simple. Health is defined as a person's ability to reach his or her vital goals ('vital goal' is defined later) given standard circumstances. If there is some vital goal that the person cannot reach in such circumstances, then he or she lacks health to some degree.

The notion of a standard circumstance must be somewhat clarified. When we ascribe an ability to a person we tacitly take our starting-point in a given standard situation or a given set of such situations. A man who is, for instance, said to be able to climb Mount Everest must succeed in doing so, if he tries, even given moderately bad assistance and moderately bad weather. But we do not require that he shall succeed, given very bad assistance or no assistance at all, or given a hurricane preventing him at the time, when he tries. The latter circumstances are not standard circumstances.

How do we determine exactly what the standard circumstances are? There is no algorithm for this. The set of standard circumstances is, if at all clearly defined, defined by choice. This choice may in its turn be dependent upon some basic evaluation on the part of the definer.

In a holistic theory of health, ability is *not* something which is characterized statistically. Ability is related to the vital goals of the individual. But what are the vital goals of man? What must a man or woman be able to do in order to be in health? Perhaps the vital goals are identical with the goals of basic human needs or perhaps they are identical with the goals consciously set by the agent.

However, these possibilities are both unsatisfactory. The first might easily lead to the following circle. According to Abraham Maslow the fulfilment of basic human needs is necessary for the maintenance of health (Maslow, 1968). Within our theory health is defined as a person's ability to realize his or her vital goals.

If vital goals are identified with the goals of basic human needs these two premises taken together give us the following circular expression: health is an ability to realize goals, the realization of which is necessary for health.

The second approach to vital goals might lead to problems with persons who have unrealistic goals. It is quite counter-intuitive to consider, for instance, a normally equipped person who has set goals which are impossible to reach as having a low degree of health. It is also strange to consider a person with very low ambitions and a very few, easily achieved, goals as having a high degree of health. (The shortcomings of these two approaches to vital goals are explored further in Nordenfelt, 1987.)

There is, however, a third possibility. The basic concept in this approach is 'happiness'. The general idea is that the vital goals of man are those states of affairs of which the fulfilment is necessary for minimal happiness. Happiness must here be understood in a general sense, covering such notions as satisfaction, contentedness and pleasure. This concept of health can be characterized in the following way (Nordenfelt, 1987):

> P is in complete health if, and only if, P is able, given standard circumstances in his or her environment, to fulfil those goals which are necessary and jointly sufficient for his or her minimal happiness.

It may seem to be a purely empirical matter whether a particular state of affairs contributes to a person's long-term happiness or not. It is our contention, however, that the concept of health thus delimited is only partially descriptive. There is an important element of valuation which comes in when we specify the limits for minimal happiness. There certainly is no purely empirical procedure by which we can discover whether someone is minimally happy. We can talk about such a procedure only when we have a standard with which to compare his or her emotional state. The setting of this standard is highly dependent on normative valuation.

4. HEALTH CARE NEED AND CHANGE

We have tried to show that evaluations enter into the assessment of health care needs on at least two levels and in a number of different respects. We argue that the ascription of needs and the ascription of health entail certain basic valuations. In general, to ascribe a need to a person presupposes that there is a goal which this person ought to approach in some respect. The choice of such a goal in its turn presupposes a valuation. Sometimes the choice of means for reaching the goal is also value-based (and not only based on causal considerations concerning efficient means for reaching the goal). Second, a holistic theory of health of the kind sketched here is a value-laden theory. The concept of a vital goal, i.e. a goal to be attained by a person in health, indicates an evaluation either on the part of the subject or on the part of some assessing person in the environment.

We have, in addition, answered a question which has been subjected to a certain amount of discussion (Springborg, 1981). Whether the concept of need contains values or not is in no way an unimportant issue. The answer has essential implications for need assessment. First, people's needs cannot be assessed only by empirical investigation if 'need' contains values—at least not until we have settled the evaluative issues. Second, it becomes necessary to take a stand on the question as to on whose values the need assessment should be based. We shall return to this issue later. We shall first deal with the factors which might influence a change in the significant value components in the concept of health care need.

4.1. Changes in the goal of need

1. When the concept of health care need is used in, for instance, the planning of health services, it becomes necessary to decide what concept of health should be used as a goal of health care need. The adoption of a holistic view of health, in such cases, may imply a change from paternalism to autonomy (see Chapter 1). It could hardly be questioned that an analytical theory of health and paternalism are well suited to one another. According to the analytical theory sketched here, a person lacks health if he or she has a disease, and he or she has a disease if an organ does not function normally. The functioning of the organ might be assessed by medical expertise only. Hence, according to an analytical theory of health it is possible that a person's health may be assessed by others without any consideration of his or her values, wants, ambitions, life-plans, etc.

   The holistic theory, on the other hand, views health as an ability to realize vital goals in a given context. The realization of vital goals is necessary for happiness. A person's happiness is to a great extent dependent on the realization of his or her wants or life-plans. (The concept of happiness is analysed in Nordenfelt, 1987.) Thus, the vital goals are in a fundamental sense influenced by an individual's values, wants, life-plans, etc. The holistic theory therefore is quite appropriate in a culture where prominence is given to individuals' autonomy.

   A change from paternalism to autonomy might not be the only change in the field of health care. In the 1980s there has also been a change from particularism to holism. Separate parts of human beings, for instance their organs, are no longer in focus in the same way as before. The whole being and its function in the social context are now emphasized. Such a change might be influenced by the same factors as the change from paternalism to autonomy—for instance, a mistrust of scientific medicine.

But some influence from other factors is conceivable. We can, for instance, notice a growing awareness that increased material welfare does not necessarily lead to increased satisfaction. We have witnessed, particularly in the last decade, an emphasizing of somewhat different values. Quality of life is a central concept in this context. The emphasis on quality of life instead of on material quantity means a change from particularism to holism.

2. The suggested concept of health, chosen from a holistic theory of health, is a dimensional one: a person may lack health to a certain degree, or a person may be more or less healthy. This means that when we intend to use such a concept of health as a goal of health care need, it becomes necessary to specify the degree of health—that is, it becomes necessary to decide upon what degree of health a person, with a need of health care, should have to reach in order for the need to be accounted as satisfied. This decision is certainly influenced by values. High ambitions with respect to health could result in an increase in the need of health care, and vice versa.

   A *rise* in the level of ambition might be influenced by the change from particularism to holism. The emphasizing of the quality of life or well-being of people may be considered as a raising of ambitions. The focusing on the whole person leads to a consideration also of mental health and social well-being.

   Furthermore, there has been in recent years a growing interest in elderly and disabled persons. New ideas about their possibilities for living a rich or decent life have led to increased demands for health. Moreover, such increased demands might also be influenced by the rise in the standard of living at large, and by the new promises generated by the development of new technology.

   However, other factors might lead to a *reduction* in ambitions—for instance, a decrease in economic resources. Such a reduction might stem from changed values. The health services compete with other urgent activities for the total resources in society. A rise in the valuation of, for instance, education or national defence might lead to a decrease in health care resources. Further, an increased use of costly life-saving therapy and growing costs for care of the elderly might be considered prohibitively expensive.

   However, a reduction in ambitions, irrespective of what factors may have influenced it, might result in a change in the acceptable level of health, and thereby a change in the health care need of the population.

4.2. Changes in the object of need

The choice of suitable means of reaching the goal of need (suitable treatment to meet the need) is perhaps in many cases an empirical issue. Medical knowledge naturally plays a principal part, as do economic considerations. Valuations might be involved in medical and economic decisions, and in some cases there might also be room for others.

We can notice a growing interest in alternative medicine, perhaps because of disappointment in the results of scientific medicine on the health of the population. But a quite noticeable change in recent decades has been the emphasis on prevention. There would seem to be two forces underlying this change. One has to do with efficiency, the other with a change from paternalism to autonomy.

There is a growing body of evidence which suggests that there are limits to what medicine could be expected to accomplish (Johnson, 1978). The major health problems facing us today—heart disease, cancer, mental illness—are problems whose causes may best be dealt with outside the realm of medicine. Insufficient physical exercise, smoking, drinking, unemployment are factors responsible for major health problems. These are factors of lifestyle and external circumstances. The proper way to deal with them is by health education or other non-medical health-promoting measures.

There seems to be, in addition, agreement that the substantial decrease in some epidemic diseases can be explained by a rise in the material conditions of living. It is possible to point to the fact that the decline in mortality and morbidity started much earlier than the expansion of medical activities. Generally, the rise in the standard of living seems, to a significant degree, to have contributed to a decline in certain diseases.

The growing insight about the importance of lifestyles for disease patterns has also resulted in an awareness of the individual's responsibility for his or her own health. We also find the view that the citizen has a responsibility for the planning and implementation of health care programmmes.

Perhaps the Declaration adopted in 1978 at Alma-Ata (Primary Health Care, 1978) is a landmark in the history of health care and health education. There it was stated that people not only have a right to participate in the planning of health care, but also have a duty to do so. It is thought that the health services should no longer filter down through a number of levels to reach the individual. There has instead been initiated, by ordinary citizens, a movement which reflects the desires of individuals to take full part in, and responsibility for, health care and health promotion. This would seem to be an excellent example of a change from paternalism to social autonomy (paternalism and autonomy are explained in Chapter 1 of this volume).

5. WHOSE VALUES SHOULD CARRY THE GREATEST WEIGHT?

The question contains the supposition that people's values or valuations differ. It is certainly a quite uncontroversial supposition. There are different interests involved in the provision of health care, and valuations seem to be connected to interests.

It is quite common, in the literature which deals with the concept of health care need, to observe the values of the patients and the values of the doctors. Some authors prefer to define the concept in terms of the doctors' opinions (Cooper, 1974). Others give the patients' and the doctors' opinions equal weight. The problem of amalgamating differing opinions in such a case is solved by a splitting of 'health care need' into two concepts, for example, felt need/normative need (Bradshaw, 1972) or perceived need/medically defined need (Mägi and Allander, 1981).

However, no one seems to consider the ordinary citizens' opinions. This might be a result of the focusing on the clinical context. It is quite possible, in such a context, that the design of care, within a given framework, concerns only patients and doctors (health personnel). The situation is different when we operate on the macro level, that is, when we try to define 'health care need' to be used in the planning of *a population's need*.

As human beings we are all vulnerable. Sooner or later we need the assistance of health services. How the health service institutions are shaped affects everybody. Ideally we should therefore all of us contribute to the political process by declaring our evaluations concerning health care. This might entail presenting what we consider to be our vital goals, but it might also entail an evaluation concerning what is a reasonable level of ambition for the health care institutions.

The question of whose values should carry the greatest weight might therefore have a simple answer—the values of the citizens. There are different methods by which those values may be considered. The Community Impression Approach is one example. The approach has three steps: interviews with key people, hard data review, and community forums (Siegel *et al.*, 1978.) But perhaps the values of citizens are best considered in a well ordered representative democracy. The settling of the valuation issues, with respect to the concept of health care need, is then a question for the political agenda.

ACKNOWLEDGMENT

We want to thank Bo Petersson, and the editors, Uffe Juul Jensen and Gavin Mooney, for valuable comments on an earlier version of our chapter.

REFERENCES

Boorse, C. (1977) Health as a theoretical concept. *Philosophy of Science* **44**, 542–73.

Bradshaw, J. (1972) A taxonomy of social need. In: *Problems and Progress in Medical Care*, McLachlan, G. (ed.). Nuffield Provincial Hospitals Trust, London.

Cooper, M. (1974) Economics of need: the experience of the British Health Service. In: *The Economics of Health and Medical Care*, Perlman, M. (ed.). Macmillan, London.
Daniels, N. (1985) *Just Health Care*. Cambridge University Press, Cambridge.
Johnson, S. C. (1978) Perspectives on the health policy process. In: *Health Care Policy in a Changing Environment*, Battistella, R. M. and Rundall, T. G. (eds), McCutchan Publishing Corporation, Berkeley.
Liss, P.-E. (1986) *A Theory of the Concept of Need*. Med. no 10/86. Department of Health and Society, Linköping University, Linköping.
Mägi, M. and Allander, E. (1981) Towards a theory of perceived and medically defined need. *Sociology of Health and Illness* **3**, 49–71.
Maslow, A. H. (1968) *Toward a Psychology of Being*, 2nd edn. D. van Nostrand, New York.
Nordenfelt, L. (1987) *On the Nature of Health*, Reidel, Dordrecht.
Primary Health Care (1978) *Report of the International Conference on Primary Health Care*. Alma-Ata, USSR, September 1978. WHO, Geneva.
Siegel, L. M., Attkisson, C. C. and Carson, L. G. (1978) Need identification and program planning in the community context. In: *Evaluation of Human Service Programs*, Attkisson, C. C. *et al.* (eds). Academic Press, New York.
Springborg, P. (1981) *The Problem of Human Needs and the Critique of Civilisation*. Allen & Unwin, London.

9

Changing Clinical Practice: A Case Study in Breast Cancer

Kaija Holli MD, Matti Hakama ScD and Gavin Mooney MA

1. INTRODUCTION

In a book concerned with changing values in health care, it is perhaps inevitable, given the antecedents of most of the chapters, that many are not concerned directly with policy change and empirical measurement thereof. Changing clinical practice can be difficult to achieve, especially in a world where being certain and perhaps more importantly where doctors desire to appear to be certain must inevitably lead to rather conservative attitudes.

Yet in cancer therapy, which is used as a case study in this chapter, it is clear that there must be uncertainty about what is the most appropriate treatment, since that is itself a value-laden concept and because the divining of what is 'most appropriate' will vary both between doctors and between patients. Some breast cancer patients will prefer to retain the breast, others to lose it. There are seldom uniquely correct methods of treatment for all even when the diagnosis is identical. There are also variations across countries, for example as indicated by Aaron and Schwartz (1984) in their comparisons of the UK and the USA. Some diseases which are quite prevalent in some countries do not apparently exist in others! For example, Clare (1989) states: 'Take the French disease spasmophilia. It is a condition that increased sevenfold in the 1970s. . . In the United States if it exists at all it is as panic disorder. In Britain it does not exist—so presumably sufferers in France might be cured simply by crossing the English Channel'.

What is done by way of medical practice is value-laden. Writing specifically of cancer, but the point could be made more generally, Stoll (1988a) states: 'Since doctors and patients often differ in their interpretation of what is good

Changing Values in Medical and Health Care Decision Making
Edited by U. J. Jensen and G. Mooney

quality of care, we must also accommodate our guidelines [for ensuring high qualities of care] to the personal preferences of each patient. Above all, we must reject a purely data-driven approach to treatment which takes little note of either patients' needs or their personal wishes'.

But, while agreeing with Stoll, we would want to suggest that the world is not quite so simple. Divining 'the personal preferences of each patient' can be very difficult and even doctors who try hard to do so may divine differently. And it is not necessarily the case, especially with terminal cancer, that patients will actually have preferences to be divined or that all patients will necessarily want their preferences to count. The individual *personalities* of patients should count; their preferences should to the extent that they, the patients, wish them to.

2. EMPIRICAL ANALYSES AND RESULTS

The studies reported here involve a research project examining the treatment and investigation of breast cancer patients in the Tampere University Central Hospital District in Finland. Aspects of these studies have been reported previously (Holli, 1987; Holli and Hakama, 1989a,b). The key foci discussed in this chapter are two: first the extent of treatment and investigation of breast cancer patients who were close to death vis-à-vis those who were not; and second the fact that in a later study period after the results of the first study had been published, the extent of some treatment and investigation of patients close to death fell.

Between 1977 and 1980 in the hospital area in question 551 patients were diagnosed as having breast cancer. Of these, 519 were followed up in a total of 8248 visits during the first 5 years. In that same 5-year period, 252 patients were diagnosed with recurrent disease; 163 of them died in that period. Thus patients were followed for either the full 5 years or up to their time of death.

Patients were classified into four groups in analysing 'last visits':

1. Last visit less than a week before death from breast cancer (called terminal stage).
2. Last visit more than a week before death from breast cancer.
3. Last visit in the 5-year period; patient alive with recurrence at the end of follow-up.
4. Last visit in the 5-year period; patient alive without recurrence at the end of follow-up.

In the second period on which we report, i.e. the period from 1 September 1987 to 31 December 1988 which followed immediately after the first publication of the results from the study period above (Holli, 1987), patients dying in the University Central Hospital Clinic in this 1987–1988 period were classified in two groups:

1. Last visit less than a week before death from breast cancer (terminal stage).
2. Last visit more than a week before death from breast cancer.

More details of the analyses in these two time periods are reported elsewhere (Holli and Hakama, 1989a,b). Here we concentrate on indicating the extent of treatment and investigation in the dying patients and the change that occurred between the two periods.

In the first period the extent of visits was much more intensive per annum for patients who died than for those who survived (8.2 visits per annum compared with 3.1).

The Karnofsky index (for which the higher the value, the better the ability of the person to function normally) at the last visit was generally much higher for the survivors with recurrent disease than for those who died. Very few of those who died were deemed at the last visit to be responding to treatment and almost invariably for these patients the disease was considered to be progressing.

There was little difference in the frequency of investigations when patients at the terminal stage were compared with others. For example, for laboratory tests, the frequency was as follows (designation of patient at last visit):

Alive without recurrence	86%
Alive with recurrence	92%
Died more than a week later	80%
Died within a week	93%

With respect to treatments it was possible to classify these as having an effect on the cancer (curative or palliative) or not. It was found that the closer the patient was to death, the greater was the cancer-related treatment. For example, chemotherapy was more than two and a half times as likely for patients within a week of death as compared with those alive with recurrent disease at the end of the 5-year follow-up period. Hormone treatment also rose in frequency as death approached—80% of patients in the terminal stage received such treatment.

This and other evidence (see Holli and Hakama, 1989a) pointed to the fact that the patients close to death were being treated and investigated more intensively than might have been expected at that terminal stage.

In the light of this study, its results and its publication in 1987 (Holli, 1987) the subsequent study was conducted (Holli and Hakama, 1989b). This covered 46 patients who died from breast cancer in the period from September 1987 to December 1988; 24 of these women died within a week of their last visit.

The results of this second study show that, while there was no change as compared with the earlier study for patients dying more than a week after their last visit, there was a substantial fall in investigations for those dying within a week of their visit. Radiological examinations fell in the University Central Hospital Clinic from 74 to 29% and laboratory tests from 92 to 58%—both statistically significant changes.

While in this second study period, as compared with the first, there were no substantial differences in the average number of treatments for either the terminal cases or those dying later than 7 days after the visit, the average intensity of treatments did fall slightly. However there was a significant decrease compared to the earlier period in the use of chemotherapy in the 1987–1988 patients who died within a week of the last visit. At the same time palliative activities aimed at relief of discomfort increased.

There is thus clear evidence that clinical practice changed between the two study periods for those patients close to death at the time of their last visit.

3. CHANGING VALUES

With respect to the first study, it might be argued that such a retrospective investigation cannot be valid because prospectively it might not be possible to form a judgment about the relative proximity of death. There are two responses we would make to this. First, while it is clearly more difficult prospectively to judge *wholly* accurately when death will occur it is far from impossible to do so fairly accurately for the types of patients involved here. Second, the existence of a prospective study, which is the only alternative, would have been known to the relevant clinicians. Such knowledge would have invalidated the study. Thus we do not accept such a criticism of the study design.

More importantly however is the fact that in our view the second study wholly vindicates our position. Treatments and investigations of patients close to death changed in the period immediately following publication of the results of the earlier study. That suggests to us at least that the knowledge of what they were doing previously led to a change in thinking by the doctors involved and that they were able to distinguish prospectively between patients in terms of their expected short-term survival, or at least to do so sufficiently well in the context of this study.

It seems reasonable to assume that there is no substantial need for conducting diagnostic investigations when the tumour is progressing, performance is poor and death from breast cancer of the patient is predictable. It can also reasonably be assumed that there is no need for intensive treatment of the cancer shortly before death. However in the first study the reverse seemed to be true. The frequency of diagnostic investigations was practically the same for patients free of recurrence and those with recurrence. Further, intensity of treatment for cancer increased the closer the patients were to death. A week or less before death there were on average 1.9 cancer treatments per patient.

The extent to which survival or quality of life can be substantially improved by information provided by diagnostic investigations during the terminal stage has to be questioned. The adverse effects, both physical and mental, caused by such activities may well outweigh any benefit expected.

It is clear that patients will receive treatment in the weeks or even days prior to death. Such a policy is assumed to be justified on the basis that some of the patients predicted to reach the terminal stage may in extreme cases live months after treatment of cancer because the treatment was effective or because the terminal event was incorrectly predicted. Such observations may be due to change, i.e. due to regression towards the mean without any real treatment effect. There is plenty of evidence that treatment of cancer does not extend the average survival at terminal stage (Powels *et al.*, 1980; Bonadonna and Valagussa, 1982; Todd *et al.*, 1983; Patel *et al.*, 1986). Even if real, such an unusual event of unexpected prolongation of life should be assessed against the adverse effects of treatment subjected to all patients. If real, there must then also be patients for whom life expectancy is shortened because of treatment.

Treatment, such as radiation, may sometimes be given for palliation. However, the most intensive increase in treatment before death in this study occurred for chemotherapy in the earlier period. When cytostatic drugs are used there are means of reducing the side-effects (Coates *et al.*, 1987). However, side-effects without any major palliation still remain and the palliation can be achieved more effectively at low cost with psychoactive or pain drugs.

Accepting and applying the cancer-related diagnosis and treatment to such an extent that adverse effects may outweigh the beneficial ones suggest that more emphasis may be being given to the cancer than to the patient. Focusing on the disease even at the terminal stage may result in the neglect of the physical and mental care of the patient. In terms of the best use of resources, less emphasis on continuing diagnostic and treatment interventions for patients at the terminal stage and more on care and comfort would seem desirable. It is most likely that this would result in increasing patients' quality of life; the impact on quantity is less certain but it can be predicted to be small or zero.

An important question relates to what the reasons are for a particular clinical practice and whether they can be changed. In the overall project and in all periods, no major changes in the distribution of treatment occurred among patients who died more than a week after the last visit. But there was a change from chemotherapy to other activities aimed at relief of discomfort of the patient among those who died a week or less after the last visit. Also the investigations at terminal stages became fewer. Therefore, in addition to the fact that the terminal stages of the breast cancer patients were capable of being adequately predicted, the results demonstrate that it is possible for substantial and rapid changes in clinical practice to occur.

The reasons for such a change remain somewhat obscure. Medicine—and that includes treatment—is accepted as functioning on a scientific basis. A reduction in the use of expensive technologies in medicine—such as chemotherapy for cancer—has been proposed on the basis of economic constraints (Stoll, 1988b; Timothy, 1988). The use of unsuccessful treatment may be due to the wishes of patients, relatives, the nurse, the doctor or other physicians or it may be a consequence of threat of legal action (Jennett, 1988).

No essential new pieces of scientific evidence on survival of patients with metastatic breast cancer appeared within this period, neither were there any changes in the resources or in the economic constraints in the clinic. The changes in clinical practice probably occurred as a result of changes in relevant value judgments. The background for such changes is not readily identifiable. The results of our first study (Holli, 1987) were originally reported in Finnish in August 1987. That report obviously created some discussion about diagnostic and treatment practices. Also in 1987–1988 the first hospice in Finland was designed and built in Tampere. The general idea on which a hospice is based may have changed attitudes more generally. The hospice itself did not influence the results: only three patients died in the hospice, all with survival of more than a week after admission. Whatever the reasons for the rapid change in the clinical practice, it is difficult to see how it could have materialized without changes in the values of the doctors responsible for the treatment of the patients in the terminal stages.

In stating that the change in clinical practice was accompanied by a change in the doctors' values, and indeed may have been caused by a change in the doctors' values, we do not mean in any way to imply that this per se is 'wrong'. It is important to recognize three key issues. First, clinical decision making does involve value judgments; second, not all clinicians will hold to the same values over time; and third, not all clinicians will exercise the same value judgments faced with the same patient/symptoms/disease stage.

In the context of the changing values of medical and health care there is a need for a much greater recognition of the extent to which individual doctors' value judgments pervade medicine. There is clear evidence in several countries for many conditions, that doctors do not treat similar patients in the same way and that this has to be in part and probably in a large part a function of the doctor (McPherson *et al.*, 1982).

In the current climate of clinical decision making it is our belief that more and more patients, albeit slowly, are becoming both more knowledgeable and more questioning about clinical practice and its effectiveness. They are not quite so ready to accept that the doctor knows best.

In the results reported above there is some evidence to support patients who might wish to question whether the doctor always knows best. If the doctors in these two periods studied were doing their best for their dying patients, it is difficult to see how we can best interpret their different actions in the two periods.

As resource constraints bite more and more on health services, there will inevitably be increasing pressure on clinicians to examine their practices for both their effectiveness and their efficiency. With respect to both, no progress can be made unless first a clear statement is made regarding what it is that is to be done effectively and efficiently. This means that clinicians must clarify what their objectives are. The studies reported here suggest that in the light of the results of the first study the clinicians involved may well have been persuaded to look more closely at what it was that they were trying to do.

In so many health services today, resource constraints are forcing consideration of effectiveness and efficiency to a greater extent than ever before. To progress further however needs clinicians to think hard about objectives and for health service policy to be devised in such a way as to provide the right climate and incentives for clinicians to reappraise their objectives. That to us is the central challenge in the current changing values in medicine and health care.

REFERENCES

Aaron, H. J. and Schwartz, W. B. (1984) *The Painful Prescription.* Brookings Institution, Washington, D.C.

Bonadonna, G. and Valagussa, P. (1982) Chemotherapy of breast cancer: current views and results. *International Journal of Radiation Oncology Biology Physics* **9**, 279–97.

Clare, A. (1989) National variations in medical practice. *British Medical Journal* **298**, 1334.

Coates, A., Gebski, V., Bishop, J. F. *et al.* (1987) Improving the quality of life during chemotherapy for advanced breast cancer. A comparison of intermittent and continuous treatment strategies. *New England Journal of Medicine* **317**, 1490–5.

Holli, K. (1987) Organization, functions and effectiveness of follow-up for breast cancer patients (in Finnish with English summary). *Acta Universitatis Tamperensis* **A 225**.

Holli, K. and Hakama, M. (1989a) Treatment of the terminal stages of breast cancer. *British Medical Journal* **218**, 13–14.

Holli, K. and Hakama, M. (1989b) Terminal stages of breast cancer, Change in a clinical practice. Submitted for publication.

Jennett, B. (1988) Medical ethics and economics in clinical decision making. In: *Medical Ethics and Economics in Health Care,* Mooney, G. and McGuire, A. (eds.) Oxford Medical Publications, Oxford, pp. 90–102.

McPherson, K., Wennberg, J. E., Hovind, D. B. *et al.* (1982) Small area variations in the use of common surgical procedures: an international comparison. *New England Journal of Medicine* **307** 1310–14.

Patel, J. K., Nemoto, T., Vezeridis, M. *et al.* (1986) Does more intense palliative treatment improve overall survival in metastatic breast cancer patients? *Cancer* **57**, 567–70.

Powels, T. J., Smith, I. E., Fort, H. T. *et al.* (1980) Failure of chemotherapy to prolong survival in a group of patients with metastatic breast cancer. Lancet **i**, 580–2.

Stoll, B. (1988a) Saying no is difficult in cancer. In: *Cost versus Benefit in Cancer Care.* Stoll, B. A. (ed.). Macmillan, London.

Stoll, B. (1988b) Balancing cost and benefit in treatment of late cancer. *British Medical Journal* **12**, 579–80.

Timothy, A. R. (1988) Cost versus benefit in non-surgical management of patients with cancer. *British Medical Journal* **297**, 471–2.

Todd, M., Shoag, M. and Cadman, E. (1983) Survival of women with metastatic breast cancer at Yale from 1920 to 1980. *Journal of Clinical Oncology* **1**, 406–8.

10

Retrenchment and Values in a Health Organization

Helge Kjersem, MD

1. INTRODUCTION

Many health services are currently facing problems in dealing with constrained resources. This has always been the case but recently this situation has become more acute because of actual cutbacks. The rationalist school argues that in these circumstances, cutbacks should be based on efficiency criteria—essentially making cuts in such a way as to minimize the fall in output or the benefit loss.

There are two forms of efficiency involved here. First, there is operational efficiency which does not challenge the objectives of the organization but attempts to retain them while meeting them at a lower cost. If this is possible, the values associated with the objectives per se remain unchanged. However, there will still be values associated with deciding which forms of resources to reduce, e.g. materials or people, doctors or cleaners. The second form of efficiency adopted by the rationalist school is that of allocative efficiency. Here the assumption is that it is not possible to maintain the previous level and mix of output. The various objectives will be competing for what resources are available. Choices then have to be made about which objectives to meet less fully than previously. Objectives are then questioned and, consequently, the values underlying these.

A common ethical principle in our society holds that any endangered human life must be saved if at all possible regardless of costs. It is almost obligatory to attempt to save a specific life at risk, even at very high costs. It is however somehow less obligatory to attempt to save a larger number of lives of anonymous individuals for the same amount of money through

---

Changing Values in Medical and Health Care Decision Making
Edited by U. J. Jensen and G. Mooney

precautions taken in advance, i.e. prevention. Decision making in health care is founded on social norms based on an aggregation of personal values in that society which are in turn related to motives, purposes and standards. These values will change over time and differ in various societies (Hofstede, 1980). Health and disease should not be looked upon solely as physical and psychological functions and dysfunctions. They are also affected by social and basic cultural interactions and the health care system per se. Health is perhaps best described as the basic perception of a human being of his or her own circumstances and quality of life.

Technically the efficiency goal of the rationalist school is to attempt to maximize the value of output whatever the level of resources. The two forms of efficiency described above assume that it is possible to define and measure the relevant output in relation to values. A major technique used is cost–benefit analysis, which normally attempts to value output in money terms. Yet it is clearly difficult to place such intangibles as the enjoyment of life itself on some measuring rod of money. Some outputs are invaluable in such terms, e.g. the prayers of religious people.

If health is based on values which reflect not only physical and psychological functions within the body but also social interactions, feelings of anxiety and uncertainty, etc., the relevant output of health services will vary both between various cultural groups and between individuals. Under the allocative form of efficiency it is therefore particularly difficult to value the benefits of health care. It follows that the value of different policies may be unstable over time as well as across different individuals and groups of individuals.

How will all of this affect the managerial and organizational requirements of a health organization in setting rationalistic efficiency goals? The study of retrenchments reported here was undertaken to examine the potential of other models for better analysing such cutback situations and therefore these models form the basis of a critique of the rational approach.

2. THE STUDY

Politicians influence our visions of the future through inter alia their economic policies. The governments in the Scandinavian countries have, over the last decade, tried to solve their countries' economic problems through retrenchments in government spending, e.g. in health care. The health care system uses much manpower and through cutbacks the governments want to decrease the number of employees in the public sector. In Denmark the government demanded 2.5–5% reductions annually in governmental hospitals and institutions in a 5-year period in the mid 1980s. I have looked at an organization structured as a professional bureaucracy with 1100 employees, of whom about 10% were highly professional academic staff who represented the powerful operational core of the organization. There was also a large support staff, plus a small administration. The work in this central national laboratory consisted of routine tests and research, delivering biomedical products such as vaccines and blood products, as well as monitoring, supervising and informing the national health care system about infectious diseases and test results. There was no direct contact with patients, so that the direct care of patients could not be used as an argument against retrenchment. The organization was structured as a professional bureaucracy, as in, for example, a hospital (Mintzberg, 1983).

I have examined three processes of decision making. The first was the 'rational way'. Here the decision makers are assumed to be fully informed; they know all the alternatives and their consequences, and have a set of well defined options for maximizing utility. They then choose in such a way as to get the most health care needed for any given amount of resources, or to get the same service for the least input (Cyert and March, 1963).

Another process of decision making is through compromising on the means of achieving different objectives. This is done through a political process (Bauer and Gergen, 1971), making compromises on different alternatives, depending on the power and ability of those involved to negotiate.

A third process can be observed in situations where options and means are difficult to determine. It may be that the link between options and means is not clear; that options do not lend themselves to explicit formulations; or that they are changing and inconsistent, perhaps thereby creating certain conflicts. Decisions can sometimes be made on a decentralized basis and/or autonomously. This is typical for anarchistic decision making processes, as in Lindblom's 'muddling through' model (Lindblom, 1959).

The retrenchments in the professional bureaucracy studied always arose in the form of sudden small cuts in the general budgets of all the departments in the organization, in relation to both materials and staff. The various departments tried constantly to avoid the cuts, primarily through different forms of argumentations. The various academic staff, e.g. physicians and chemical engineers, tried to strengthen their own positions of power in the organization. Tensions arose between colleagues and departments, and between various groups of workers. The small annual retrenchments had a short time-horizon: the organization always hoped for 'business as usual next year'. The relatively small administration, which is normally seen in health organizations such as this one as functioning as a professional bureaucracy, tried to avoid conflicts by demanding several smaller, overall retrenchments throughout the organization.

Explicit priorities were not set across the different departments during the 5-year period of observation. During the first year it was possible to keep the same level of activity, but only at the expense of postponing new and more ambitious projects. The retrenchments did not seem to relate to any well defined objectives or mechanisms in the organization. Services were decentralized to the county hospitals, production of services and commodities were somewhat rationalized, the levels of service output were kept unchanged.

In more recent years the academic staff have started to become demoralized and the climate among employees has worsened because of the increased workload. Some departments have started to function inefficiently because of the lack of setting of priorities. Cutbacks were made more or less equally across the different departments throughout the period. The academic staff tried to retain their autonomy in their work, which was possible because of the complexity of the different working processes. The administration had the possibility of influencing the organization through their control over resources. However, lacking knowledge and perhaps information of the working processes, it seemed to be impossible to make the cutbacks in any way which could be linked to well defined options and means.

3. SOME IMPLICATIONS

There are different kinds of decision making in different situations, e.g. under various political processes and organizations. The lack of priority setting even after several years of retrenchments in this health organization seemed to indicate that the idea of pursuing rational decision making within a professional bureaucracy may not be possible or at least was not possible in this instance.

It should be noted that anarchistic processes of decision making without well defined options and means are not the same as anarchy. Lindblom's 'muddling through' model suggests several small steps involving a process of trial and error. Such a process does not necessarily lead to a bad outcome.

The use of another anarchistic model of decision making in a health organization, the 'garbage can' model (Cohen *et al.*, 1972), could also be used to regulate whose values count. In this model the processes are divided into four parts, which could be combined and monitored differently: the problems; the solution of the problems; the number of participants, and the frequency of meetings or events. The events are the 'garbage cans' into which various solutions, participants and problems are thrown. If the right combination occurs or is considered to have occurred, decisions can then be made.

However, during times of retrenchment the ideas of political decision makers do not seem to be founded only on economic calculations. Such calculations seem also to be used by the bureaucrats to test the validity of these ideas. If the economic prognosis is shown not to be valid, the economists will point to the political ideas as being proved wrong. If the bureaucrats' economic calculations are used to test the validity of political ideas—such as solidarity, taking care of those who suffer, equal access to health care, etc.—the economists can show that these ideas are wrong. This change towards economic rationality during retrenchments in health care has somewhat overshadowed political values. However, rationality is also controlled by values (Simon, 1957) and will change over time.

The values underlying the economic theories adopted by bureaucrats should be made explicit for the political decision makers, who should be listening to and understanding the values of their voters. Political ideas should not be justified on the basis of economic prognoses and theories. Moral values have to be taken into consideration, particularly in health care decision making.

The academic staff of this professional bureaucracy seemed to be the key part of the organization. By controlling information, knowledge and skills, they were able to persuade, induce or coerce others to follow certain courses of actions.

Physicians are, through their personal qualities but also through a high level of consensus in the society, viewed as indispensable to the health care system. This basic cultural assumption gives the physicians a powerful position strategically. Through their knowledge and skills and through their control of channels of communication to the bureacratic decision makers, they have the power to influence decisions on what is needed in health care.

The administrative decision makers can control resource allocation. However, in health care the bureaucratic administrator will have difficulties in making rational decisions based on efficiency criteria. The rational decision maker will lack the information either to decide which resources to reduce during retrenchments if objectives are to remain unchanged or to attempt to maintain the level and value of the outputs whatever the level of resources.

The administrator or manager of a health organization, faced with retrenchments, should therefore have professional skills combined with administrative skills to achieve the most efficient economic solutions, taking the values of the society, as well as the staff in the organization and the customers/patients, into account.

This is an important consideration, especially as physicians are becoming more specialized and have lost some of their privileged position as omnipotent doctors surrounded by mysticism in their job. Attempting to make themselves indispensable through specialization can be questioned by an administrator who has both professional and administrative skills. The administrator can limit the doctors' power in the hierarchy through isolation.

The power of doctors is also diminishing because of the advances in biomedical skills of nurses and other health care workers, who are in a stronger position to exercise discretion through the nature of their jobs. They interpret ordinations of physicians and execute particular parts of the decision makers' policy, using their own personal discretion.

The greater knowledge of patients gives them greater power, as they are no longer willing just to accept the 'take it or leave it' attitude in health care. This has led to a greater demand for autonomy in health care in the last few decades. Involving the patients more in decision making in health services will also provide a more immediate feedback and monitoring of the results, thereby leading to more incentives and pressures for improvements. Involving the patients and/or relatives in health services during retrenchments can reduce the demand for manpower as seen in other service industries (Normann, 1983), e.g. relatives can be educated to take part of the physical and mental training of patients; groups of patients can educate each other under supervision (high blood pressure groups, overweight groups, etc.). The level of education has been increasing generally in society and the change in values and scepticism towards authority have increased the interest in democratic decision making in the bureaucracy. To meet the needs of the consumers of health services—the patients—it is better to involve them more emotionally and intellectually in the production of such services.

The most important resources in any health organization are the staff involved in providing the services. During retrenchments it is important to have some form of personnel policy for the members of the organization, to boost feelings of security and to reduce anxiety, to keep them motivated and working together in the interest of the institution. It is important for the members of the organization to be fully informed and to be able to trust the administration to work efficiently for common objectives and to support the values underlying these. The challenge of retrenchments might then be met more enthusiastically, involving the members in the anarchistic processes of decision making in order to change the beliefs, attitudes and values in the organization through a more complex educational strategy. The top manager should therefore be trusted by the professionals as a professional, but a professional with management skills. The organization will not survive retrenchments through economic theories alone, but through the members' consensus of objectives and the values underlying them.

During periods of retrenchment the administration will try to obtain more control over the professionals. As shown here, this will result in demotivation and resistance among these staff members. The result does not seem to have been increased economic efficiency. It is therefore important to promote a combination of professional and management skills at the very top of any health organization. Then anarchistic decision making processes can be monitored together with political and rational decision making in various situations to mobilize the human resources in the organization. The resultant motivations and visions among staff can then deal better with governmental cutbacks.

4. IMPLICATIONS FOR RATIONALITY

As shown here, rational economic theories will have difficulty in operating in a health organization because of the power of the knowledge and skills of the professionals. However, the professionals will not necessarily simply protect their power and privileges. Their professional and human values can be mobilized through a leadership which can be trusted to respect these values. The changes imposed on the organization by the governmental retrenchments can then strengthen it and make a better prognosis for survival of the organization in the longer run.

Does this mean that the rational model cannot be applied to health care organizations? The answer here seems to be yes—and no.

It cannot be successfully applied if it is assumed that the application will by itself create efficiency. There are few, at least when they understand the notion of efficiency, who would want to argue against it in principle. The problems are partly on the methodology per se of pursuing efficiency, particularly in the formalized version of cost–benefit analysis. Here the measurement and valuation problems are obvious—particularly when we are dealing with health organizations whose outputs are reduced mortality, decreased suffering and pain and other key intangible concerns which often seem to defy measurements. Although these problems are at least recognized by the rationalist school, it is the operational and management problems of the real world that the rationalists too often ignore.

It may well be that an efficient organization may be a worthwhile goal, but it may not fit in with the goals of individuals or groups of individuals within the organization. Private goals and organizational goals often conflict, and responses to change from retrenchment will often appear to be irrational. The lack of fixed goals and means for individuals in the organization during retrenchment will therefore favour an anarchistic process of decision making as described above.

There is no strictly right or strictly wrong way of making decisions, but various processes of decision making will function at different levels and in different situations. However, when the goals of the organization conflict with the goals of individuals or groups within the organization, the underlying values of these goals will also be in conflict. This does not mean that rationalism fails and has to be replaced in all situations, rather that we should have in mind that rational decision making is controlled by values and can change in its nature and its recommended actions over time. It is this dynamic view of rationalism that makes the use of rational decision making in health care a very real challenge.

REFERENCES

Bauer, R. A. and Gergen, K. J. (eds.) (1971) *Study of Policy Formation*. The Free Press, New York.

Cohen, M. D., March, J. G. and Olsen, J. P. (1972) A garbage can model of organizational choice. *Administrative Science Quarterly*, **17**, 1–25.

Cyert, R. M. and March, J. G. (1963) *A Behavioral Theory of the Firm*. Prentice-Hall, Englewood Cliffs.

Hofstede, G. (1980) *Culture's Consequences: International Differences in Work Related Values*. Sage Publication, Beverly Hills.

Lindblom, C. E. (1959) The science of 'muddling through'. *Public Administration Review* **XIX**, 79–88.

Mintzberg, H. (1983) *Structures in Fives: Designing Effective Organizations*. Prentice-Hall, New Jersey.

Normann, R. (1983) *Service Management*. Bedriftsøkonomisk forlag, Oslo.

Simon, H. A. (1957) *Administrative Behaviour* (2nd edn.). Macmillan, New York.

11

Hungarian Health Care: A Challenge to Medical Values?

Tamas Angelus, PhD

1. INTRODUCTION

As the economies of the industrialised world have expanded in the period since the end of World War II, there has been a tendency for health services to grow even faster and with them their costs. In particular it has been the hospital sector that has expanded.

Such development has been supported by the rapid adoption by health services of the results of scientific and technological advances. Ultrasonic equipment, laser technology and various computerised systems have quickly become 'routine'. Such new technology provides a lot of information never known previously about the functions of the human body, thereby helping to make more accurate and faster diagnosis of various symptoms.

These new technologies however not only assist in addressing existing needs, they also result in expanded needs. They provide more information. They are normally less problematical than the technologies they replace; so they are used more. The spread of ultrasound in pregnancy is a case in point. It is easy; it is safe; it is used. Costs are not seen as a problem at the clinical level—indeed they are not seen at a clinical level. Diagnoses are made faster and better, often it seems because they can be made faster and better. Symptoms are more often and more quickly picked up even if no better patient management is clearly available.

There is the feeling of if it's there, we should have access to it. The technological imperative is strong. Doctors' training and their values push them to do the best they can for their patients. The best becomes associated—sometimes, but only sometimes rightly—with the most advanced

Changing Values in Medical and Health Care Decision Making
Edited by U. J. Jensen and G. Mooney

technology. Yet the values underlying health care as a social institution cannot sustain these technology-led values of medicine.

Earlier and more accurate diagnoses are not always followed by the successful treatment of the disease(s). The possibilities for improved health have not increased as fast as those for the diagnosis of the problems.

Technological development has increased the costs of health services. But the effectiveness of these services has not increased pro rata.

Some countries—the richer ones—are better placed to sustain and finance new technological leaps forward. But medicine is international and quickly the new technology of the richest becomes their routine; and pressure mounts on the poorer countries to advance their technological frontiers.

This chapter examines this issue in the specific context of Hungary, a country which has witnessed many changes in recent years, in its society and economy, in health care and in health. It exemplifies some of the problems that arise when medical values are not sustained by social values.

2. HUNGARY

Hungary is a Mid-East European country with over 10 million inhabitants. It is an agrarian–industrial country and a member of the Warsaw pact. In the last few years new reforms have been started both in the economy as well as in politics.

Health care in Hungary is the responsibility of the state. Between the two World Wars professional medical care was available to only a small minority of the Hungarian population. Only 31% of the population were entitled to free health care through sickness insurance. After World War II, high priority was given to organising health care for the whole population. By the mid 1960s 85% of people were covered and by 1975 practically 100% were insured.

The 1972 Public Health Act provided that, as from 1975, each citizen was entitled as a right to free medical care at that level required by his or her disease and/or condition and according to the current state of the art of medicine.

The principle of progressive patient care which is endorsed in Hungary means in practice that patients are referred to that particular level of health care delivery system where the most appropriate care can be delivered. Such health care delivery has five levels:

1. The *primary health care* level: this includes district GPs' services, district paediatricians' services and industrial health services.
2. The *municipal* level: municipal hospitals providing in- and outpatient care for basic specialties.
3. The *county* level: county hospitals providing specialised care in a wider range of specialties.

4. The *regional* level: regional centres (in seven regions of the country) providing highly specialised care (e.g. heart surgery, renal dialysis, special diagnostics), and sophisticated health care in the different medical specialties.
5. The *state* level: national institutes of health providing highly specialised medical care.

Another specific and important feature of the Hungarian health care system is integration, in the course of which the previously independent network of clinics providing outpatient care has been combined with hospitals with respect to organisation, function and finance in order to ensure a more efficient division of labour, a better mix between inpatient and outpatient care, as well as a more effective utilisation of resources.

Hungary is faced with the problem outlined in the introduction to this chapter: it seeks and to a large extent obtains modern, expensive technology. But in the Hungarian context (and in other relatively poor countries) this is clearly not the most efficient way to deploy the scarce health resources available.

Resources are limited. But what is then very important and of interest is their distribution. In other words there is a need to establish priorities: which fields, tasks, goals should be developed and financed? For which are resources not enough? Planning and setting priorities cannot of course totally bridge the gap between what is demanded and how far resources will go. But at least an effort can be made, or at least should be made, to give priority to those goals that society values most highly.

This rationing phenomenon is a characteristic of all health care systems in all countries. But for countries like Hungary the problems of planning are exacerbated by the presence of expensive technologies and ineffective results.

Such circumstances demand that the values of society rather than medical ones come more to the fore as the dominating ones in health care. This chapter discusses this issue against the background of already changing values but in particular of the recognition that they are changing in the wrong direction.

As an example, let us take the case of the computerised tomography (CT) scanner. This is a modern, non-invasive, safe form of X-ray. It can provide very precise diagnoses about the human body, for example in the early detection of tumours. It is very expensive.

Such diagnoses must be or at least ought to be followed by adequate therapy. There are then two problems. The therapeutic methods do not always exist; where they do, they cannot always be afforded.

What is the current situation in Hungary? We have the diagnoses (and therefore the patient has the knowledge of his or her—possibly fatal—disorders). We have paid a lot to get the knowledge. But we cannot help the patient! Such a situation has to be unethical. It is an inefficient use of (limited) resources. Other better ways of using the resources are thereby forgone; for example in the care of the elderly, where the benefit could be greater, allowing more patients to achieve a higher quality and standard of life.

For relatively poor countries, the question then becomes very real: why use (limited) resources on such very expensive technologies? It is a fact that Hungary at present has four CT scanners and one nuclear magnetic resonance (NMR) imager.

Clearly I can do no more than estimate the results of spending these resources in another way. What is clear is that the benefit of that reallocation would do more good than is the case under the current allocation pattern. But professionals want to, are driven to invest in advanced technology. They do not want to be left behind in the technological race: technology takes on a value in itself.

Of course it is relevant to go beyond the health care field and ask whether, even allowing for low efficiency in the health care sector, resources might not be better spent on health care than in other parts of the economy, given how poorly the rest of the economy is performing. Such poor performance has resulted in a falling standard of living for most of the population. The economy lacks investment which puts a brake on development, which could otherwise increase the standard of living and perhaps in turn allow increased spending on health care.

Such a proposition—invest in the economy now so that there may be more to invest in health care in the future—sounds fine. But it excludes the interests of the present population. Even if it could be proved that it would result in better health for future populations, it is simply not possible to persuade the present population to agree to such an approach to planning. They see the sacrifice today as too great. Further there is scepticism about how bright the future would be. There could be no guarantee either that the increased investment in the economy would yield large returns, or that if these large returns did occur, they would be devoted to the improvement of health.

3. THE HEALTH SITUATION IN HUNGARY

The health status of populations is often measured by age-specific mortality rates. These improved rapidly in Hungary in the first decade after World War II. Thereafter there was a significant increase in mortality rates. The first 20 years after the war were characterised by a decrease in infectious diseases, followed by an increase in non-infectious diseases, with a high mortality rate in the 40–69-year-old male population.

In the same period health services grew apace. For example, the number of GPs' offices increased by 33%, and outpatient consulting hours at polyclinics by nearly 50%. The number of hospital beds increased by 40%. (At present we have 97.4 beds per 10 000 population.) There was a substantial growth in the numbers of health service personnel (a 10% increase for physicians; 50% for nurses). The number of physicians is currently 28.5 per 10 000 population; the number of nurses is 6.6 per 10 000 population. Health expenditure increased by 470%, while the national income rose by only 320%.

Parallel with the changes in the economy as a whole in the late seventies, living standards first failed to continue to grow and then actually fell. The population was faced with taking on extra jobs if they were to maintain their standard of living, resulting in a reduction in their leisure time. As a consequence, stress and the consumption of alcohol and tobacco increased.

There was a significant movement of the population. In the last 25 years the population of Budapest (the capital) has increased by 15%, and of other cities by 40%, while the numbers living in villages have fallen by 13%.

While the number of marriages decreased by 17% between 1960 and 1985, the number of divorces rose by 77%. In 1960, 55% of divorced couples had children. This proportion in 1985 was 67%. In 1985 52% of women over 60 years of age were widows as a consequence of the increased mortality rate of middle-aged men.

The changing family pattern is also characterised by the one-child model families. A negative demographic trend has developed in the last few years.

The educational level increased quickly, but a rather high proportion involved on-the-job training which caused changes in lifestyle and stressful situations.

Morbidity across the different social groups differs markedly. According to a recent study, there is a 10-year difference in the morbidity pattern between the highest and lowest qualified social groups. For example, the same morbidity pattern is seen in the 30–39-year age group of unskilled workers as in the 40–49-year-old managers.

Alcohol consumption increased from 6.1 to 11.6 litres of pure alcohol per capita per annum between 1960 and 1985. The death rate from cirrhosis of the liver was 0.89 per 10 000 in 1960, 2.8 per 10 000 in 1980 and 4.3 per 10 000 in 1985.

There has been an increase in the consumption of tobacco in recent decades. It is estimated that 50% of men and 19% of women aged over 15 are smokers. Cigarette consumption in 1970 was 22.5 thousand million and 23.2 in 1985. The mortality caused by cancer of the respiratory system was 23.0 per 100 000 in 1960, 65.5 per 100 000 in 1980 and 88.1 per 100 000 in 1986.

Violent deaths are also very frequent. The rate for traffic accidents in 1986 was 21.1 per 100 000, and in non-traffic accidents 56 per 100 000. The rate of fatal suicides was 44.4 per 100 000 in 1985.

In Hungary where the health status of adults, particularly the male population, has worsened, there is thus a negative correlation with the development of the health services.

4. VALUES IN DEVELOPMENT

The problems and 'diseases' of health care are not understandable in themselves. They need to be considered in the context of the political and social development of a country.

Improvement in health services is only possible if there is a more general improvement in the country as a whole. The enormous improvement in health that is the utopia endorsed as supposedly a possible future reality in the 38 targets of WHO/EURO (WHO, 1985) is exposed as no more than a slogan.

The situation regarding the state of health in most countries in the world—including East Europe—shows however that the targets are unrealistic. It is therefore essential, at least in the context of Hungary, that the national programme should lower these utopian goals if they are to have any genuine possibility of being achieved.

Health promotion is based on the slogan: 'The principal value is man'. Health is a key element in human dignity. But these are empty words when billions are starving and millions face death from starvation. The distress, the starvation are more humbling than sickness and affect and diminish not only the victims but also those who look upon them, even if they themselves are not threatened. Yet in a world in which so much power and energy are wasted through science and high technology on the production and maintenance of weapons, we have to address the question: in an apparently senseless world, how much sense is there in creating widespread public health programmes?

There is no doubt that much thought has gone into the production of the 38 WHO targets and that these reflect current knowledge about the health status of all Europe. But the targets do not take sufficient account of the differences between countries, the important differences in the fields of economic, of political, of social and of health development.

Many of the targets of WHO derive their modus vivendi from a value system which emphasises prevention. That is fine; but it is not enough. They do not embrace the necessary and justified criticism of the prime current contender for scarce resources, namely curative medicine. More resources may be attracted for the advancement of health, but if they are not, then more resources for prevention can only come about at the expense of curative medicine. That needs to be stated firmly. The WHO targets do not do so.

The current and past dominance of the values which have resulted in emphasis being placed on the somatic view must be challenged.

The psychosomatic aspects of medicine need to be given greater priority. High technology medicine has to be seen for what it is: all too often all too expensive for what it delivers to the patient's health status. And it is that status that should count, not the technological status of the equipment used.

Any analysis of the morbidity and mortality patterns and trends of European countries since World War II shows that the greatest improvements have been in those countries with a so-called 'welfare state'. Unfortunately the East European (socialist) countries—among them Hungary—cannot show such advantageous results in these respects. In 1960 mortality rates in Finland were worse than in Hungary; by 1982 Finland was one of the best placed in Europe in these respects while Hungary's position was among the worst.

Various health indicators after World War II and into the 1960s, in the period of extensive development of health services, improved in Hungary. But this progress stopped and today there is none.

The WHO targets highlight the fact that the poor and even deteriorating health situation of the Hungarian population cannot improve without intersectoral collaboration. It is a task that the health service alone cannot tackle successfully.

An analysis made recently by the Hungarian Ministry of Health emphasises that we have the worst mortality record in Europe, which must also reflect our poor morbidity. Partly this is a result of the unhealthy lifestyle of our people. The survey indicates that despite the apparent development of health services, the health situation of the population is deteriorating.

Diseases of the circulatory system, neoplasms and accidents are particularly problematic. It is these which give rise to our high mortality rate. It is or ought to be a key concern of the whole society to improve this situation. To do so a health policy is required which covers the whole of society, which emphasises that concerns for health ought to pervade all our working and living conditions, and which in the interests of all (individuals as well as organisations) would be based on the promotion and improvement of health and the prevention of disease.

Looking back at the way Hungary has developed, at the extensive industrialisation in the last decades, it seems that often the fundamental principle has been forgotten: 'The principal value is man'. It is necessary to achieve radical changes in the realisation of this principle in terms of humanising both work and the economy more generally. It is not enough to aspire to shorter working hours, to speed up production only to increase its intensity. It needs new 'humanised' technology. Health promotion is not a reality and will not become a reality until such thinking pervades all aspects of our daily lives. We cannot put health in a separate compartment. The humanisation of production and of the economy should mean that the economy is for man and not man for the economy.

The democratic organisation of work; the fair distribution of income; social security; the availability of training: all are elements in this humanisation process. Only in this way can the stress of daily living, so harmful to health, be diminished.

There is furthermore a need for change at the everyday, cultural level. This development would have its impact at the level of daily work, the effective use of leisure time, on eating habits and other aspects of lifestyle.

Environmental protection needs promotion. It must be understood that the (mis)use of the environment has only very short-term advantages. It must be understood that we are part of the environment and its misuse turns against us. Here again the basic principle must be that of prevention. Avoiding ecological harm is both easier and cheaper than repairing the damage afterwards.

To eradicate the problems of our social and health policy, widespread social and health reforms are necessary. The first stage of this reform programme is to ensure that in future these formerly separated fields are integrated.

The diseases which are increasing today stem from a psychosocial background. It is simply not possible to deal with them with medical tools alone.

It is also clear that social problems, diseases, and social disorders are not eliminated through conventional 'social security'. We have lived with these problems for a long time. The tool of optimal influence here is again prevention. Preventive social policy and preventive health policy are to be promoted not only because they are effective but because prevention of social problems/diseases is also cheaper compared with ex post facto repair and treatment.

At all levels of health services there is a need for an up-to-date, organised system of delivery of care in the interests of more effective and efficient work. The primacy of primary care is a slogan that is now 10 years old. In European societies however current practice is quite otherwise. 'Primary care' in practice is basic medical care. This is fine. The problem is that this basic care does not work well enough. Too many patients look for 'better care' at higher levels of the health care system.

5. MEDICAL VALUES VS. SOCIAL VALUES

In recent years, the extensive development of medical services has resulted, in theory at least, in a policy of progressive patient care. Considerable attention has been paid to institutional care. Sometimes this policy has resulted in relative over-provision of a service. Too much was spent on hospitals and other institutions. The theory of this development was that 'better and better' (equipped) services give better and better care, resulting in better and better health.

Yet in this same period the health of the population has deteriorated. There has been an increase in mortality caused by cardiovascular diseases. Mortality generally among the middle-aged male population in Hungary has increased significantly. (Unfortunately this tendency characterises most East European countries.) Further, the economic crisis in Hungary in the last few years has meant that the standard of living has in general decreased and this has hit the elderly particularly badly.

The community is now faced with a new phenomenon: poverty. And it is well known that poverty has its own health consequences: for example, tuberculosis. The prevalence of this disease is again increasing. The relative (and sometimes the absolute) poverty of the whole economy is too often accompanied by the polluting of the environment and, inevitably, its harmful effects on health.

In the battle or conflict between medical and social values, the medical values have to date won. That cannot be allowed to continue.

East Europe and with it Hungary are changing. *Glasnost* and *perestroika* point to reforms in very many aspects of society. In Hungary the need for change in policy and more fundamentally in values in health and social policy is very great. The medical values of the past have failed us. The new political values must allow substantial reform in health and social care. And there is a desperate need to do better, as earlier sections of this chapter have attempted to reveal.

The detail of change is yet to be worked out. But there is agreement that more experimentation with new forms of economic organisation is needed as well as a greater acceptance of the desirability of new incentive mechanisms on the supply side. In health care, the state will surely retain its overall responsibility for basic care for all citizens but it must now ensure that the values underpinning that basic care reflect better those of consumers and potential consumers—that is, social values—and less those of medicine, as has happened in the past.

Beyond that basic level of care, the current view would seem to point to some fee for service insurance-based system. Just how this would be developed in practice is not yet clear. Certainly we in Hungary would want to learn from the experiences in other countries with such mixed systems. And we would want to keep health rather than medicine centre-stage in choosing the Hungarian method.

That means inter alia a broadly based health programme, including not just health but social care. In the last two or three years two-digit inflation has hit many badly, but especially the elderly pensioners. The real value of pensions has fallen and with it the need for social support has increased. But it is not just the elderly who suffer. The young for example cannot get adequate housing.

The way out and the way forward are clear: the government must stop supporting inefficient sectors of the economy, develop measures to promote economic growth and thereby provide more resources for health and social services.

But life is not so simple. Such plans are easy to state: their realisation is inevitably slow.

Beyond these more macro-orientated general problems, I think that the current health care system can also be improved from within, especially in terms of improved, more flexible management of health services and especially hospitals. Through better management can come greater efficiency and more and better health, even with the existing level of resources.

But such economic, political and management changes need a change of heart and a change of values on the part of the doctors and of the patients if they are to succeed. The doctors must accept the need for economic values in good patient care—that such values stress the need for doing better in the interest of patients—and the patients must learn to trust the health services to provide the health care they seek.

REFERENCE

WHO (1985) *Targets for Health for All*. WHO Regional Office for Europe, Copenhagen.

12

Medical Malpractice Phenomena: Signals for Changing Medical and Health Care Values

Inger Brødsgaard, MD and Rod Moore, DDS, MA

1. TOWARD A DEFINITION OF MEDICAL MALPRACTICE PHENOMENA

Medical malpractice (MM) has been defined in a 1986 report from the United States' Government's General Accounting Office (GAO; 1986) as 'bad, wrong, or ''injudicious'' treatment of a patient by a medical professional resulting in injury, unnecessary suffering, or death because of ignorance, carelessness, lack of skill, or criminal intent'.

But it is more than that. It is a multidimensional phenomenon influenced by political, social, commercial, legal and economic forces within societies. Changes in occurrence and variations in the nature of this phenomenon are considered to be symptoms of imbalance in one or more of these societal forces.

In this chapter by describing the systems created in response to the phenomenon in our native countries (the USA and Denmark) as well as in the UK, we see questions arise, ideas emerge and personal and societal values evolving and transforming the doctor–patient relationship. We see patterns of differing concepts of autonomy as reinforced by the different catalysts; in one model (the USA) the lawyers are catalysing the change whereas in another (Denmark) the state is the catalyst.

Changing Values in Medical and Health Care Decision Making
Edited by U. J. Jensen and G. Mooney

We use the abbreviation MM throughout the chapter and refer to the phenomenon as either:

1. The actual happening of medical incompetence as within the above definition, or:
2. The more complex phenomenon as a whole, the MM here used in combination with the word 'phenomenon'.

We focus on doctors here, since the majority of serious injuries are caused by doctors, although dentists, nurses and other health care personnel can also give maltreatment.

MM has been an unavoidable part of modern western health care involving legislators, lawyers, economists and health care personnel, but only in recent years has the public's focus on the subject made the MM claim response more assertive.

What is the problem? How big is it? Is there really a problem or is it a natural societal development? These simple questions lead to complex answers which we begin to address in this chapter. We do so from our backgrounds as researchers and practising clinicians.

2. THE PHENOMENON IN NUMBERS

In the USA with 235 million people and about 550 000 doctors, the phenomenon of MM has existed for about as long as the Constitution (1789), and has increased exponentially over the years (Sabiston, 1985). There was an average of 14 074 cases filed in 1975 and 1976; over 42 000 in 1983; 73 468 cases in 1984 and finally close to 95 000 in 1986 (Coleman, 1989). Of the claims filed in 1984, 31 782 (43%) were settled in favour of the plaintiff. A total of $2.6 billion was paid out from the insurance companies in awards; obstetricians and surgeons were responsible for the highest individual awards (GAO, 1987a).

In the mid 1970s with the first substantial upsurge, many malpractice insurance companies, unprepared for the rise in the number of claims, fled the market. A few companies remained, but raised their malpractice insurance rates dramatically, in some states by as much as 300% in one year. This has evened out again over the years so that the average increase statewide was 17.5% in 1988, down from 22% the year before.

Consequently physicians then began to practise a more defensive type of medicine and many local state regulations put limits on claims, awards and legal fees. Today these safeguards have often been declared unconstitutional, judged upon a few exceptional cases (GAO, 1986).

Thus, the phenomenon continues to grow, unchecked by lawmakers. Today, for example, it is difficult in some states of the USA such as Florida, Alabama and Nevada for women to find a physician to deliver babies. In

September 1987, it was reported that 12% of all American obstetricians had stopped delivering babies and that more than half of Alabama's counties were without obstetric care. In California and rural Nevada over half of all family practitioners have given up obstetrics (Mayer, 1987). Another example: most American doctors think twice and usually refuse to handle chance emergency situations, such as automobile accidents outside their clinics, for fear of being sued.

In Denmark, where there are 5 million residents and 14 000 doctors, the numbers of filed claims have climbed steadily from 113 around 1970, to 1093 in 1988.

But why have patients, lawyers, lawmakers and insurance companies not responded until recently? Are, for example, doctors becoming more incompetent or has society only recently become more aware of the incompetent minority of doctors that has always existed? How has this affected the doctor–patient relationship in general? What are reasonable ways to respond to the situation?

3. DESCRIPTION OF THE PHENOMENON IN THE USA

The MM legal system, as developed in the USA was originally designed to perform two functions: to deter medical incompetence or negligence and to compensate its victims (Danzon, 1984).

Settlements are made out of court in 90% of cases. In court, doctor peer review panels and expert witnesses testify, and a jury makes the final judgment. The attorney is paid a percentage or a contingency fee, commonly from 30 to 40% of any award or settlement (GAO, 1987a). A case lost means no money for the lawyer.

In most states physicians are required to have malpractice insurance by law (GAO, 1987a). The malpractice insurance companies have international or foreign reinsurers (such as, e.g. Lloyd's of London), which help to relieve the economic up and down swings of MM claims and thus influence insurance company policies and premiums (GAO, 1986).

The problem of MM is dealt with in all levels of the American society, including the highest political level, with the Senate discussing bills now and then in an attempt to build up some general constitutional rules regarding how to handle this phenomenon. At the same time every state in the USA is confronted with different sides of this complex situation and have to act now, which has prompted each state to create their own local set of solutions and restrictions.

Everybody in the American health care system and most people in touch with it have been affected in some way by the huge complex phenomenon of MM. It seems to have a life of its own, where each group has a different perspective, which contributes to the whole process.

Patients' perspective

The patient is alone, up against two mighty and authoritative professions—medical and legal. Even if the individual wins the case, the lawyer wants 30–40%, maybe even 50% of the award.

Going to the doctor has become very expensive: the doctor requests more tests, charges higher fees, and spends less time with the patient. In some cases the doctor asks for the patient's signature as proof that the patient has been informed of the risks of the treatment in order to avoid a lawsuit in case something goes wrong (Huttmann, 1981). For the same reason some physicians even refuse to treat a patient if the individual is poor, or maybe even just black or hispanic. And sometimes the patient may ask: 'Is he good enough, competent enough?', knowing that some doctors barred from practising in one location move to another area to practise (GAO, 1987b). With all this, patients have begun to question their belief in the doctor as the unrockable authority figure. And as a patient it is difficult to understand why 'bad doctors' would be protected by their colleagues.

Doctors' perspective

Rocketing MM insurance premiums, higher costs of new technology and the risk of being sued have forced the doctors to practise more expensive so-called 'defensive medicine', which includes more tests, refusals to perform certain procedures and greater selectivity of new patients and has also forced new doctors to choose low-risk specialties. Doctors had for years accepted their own definitions of 'reasonable risk' or the chance of something going wrong for a patient, in spite of every possible precaution. Now these definitions are questioned by lawyers who often may lack knowledge of the context of medical practice. Doctors feel lawyers have created a monopoly and that they are inviting the patients in to play the 'sue your doctor' lottery—the so-called 'lottery syndrome'.

Health care is becoming a big business, in which physicians feel they must emphasize price more than quality, due to third-party pressures. The values of the physician–patient trust and what is best for the patient are suffering from outside economic forces (Relman, 1987).

It is a minority of incompetent doctors who are the reason for the very high insurance rates. Examples are: 6.6% of Maryland's doctors were responsible for 93.7% of the claims paid from 1976 to 1986; 3% of doctors in Florida were responsible for 48% of the claims paid in a 10-year period and one doctor had 34 paid claims (Winkenweider and Ball, 1988). It is only recently that doctors began to see the necessity of stricter discipline of their incompetent colleagues (GAO, 1987b).

Lawyers' perspective

For American lawyers the MM phenomenon is good business in which they can make a lot of money and, from their perspective, improve the health care system, while preventing medical negligence at the same time by economic deterrence.

The lawyers thus often blame doctors' carelessness and malpractice insurance companies for the growing MM problem, but do not see it as a problem which they cannot deter with amoral legal knowledge.

Insurance companies' perspective

On the other hand, malpractice insurers, such as St Paul Companies, the nation's largest MM insurer, blame the dramatic rise in insurance rates on increased claims against doctors and more costly settlements (Appleby, 1987). They state that MM insurance is an extraordinarily difficult type of insurance because one never knows how much a claim is going to be, and sometimes cases are strung out for years and years, creating an unreliable cyclical nature of profits. For these reasons St Paul stopped insuring new physicians as of January 1986 (Appleby, 1987).

The central problem of MM from the insurers' perspective is that patients have their expectations too high; also, in court the jury tends to sympathize with patients rather than to be rational and objective (Physicians Insurance Company of Ohio, personal communication).

As a result of these widely differing perspectives, a vicious circle of MM is created. It has become a business phenomenon, where the main drive is no longer justice or better health care, but money. Thus one should ask oneself: is the MM phenomenon beneficial to the US health care system? Is it a necessary development? And if not, is it yet another catalysing factor that inflates health care cost and could contribute to bankruptcy of the system regardless of good or evil intention? There appears to be a problem here, but each group either blames the other or denies the problem's existence. American doctors have even begun to discuss national health insurance or socialized medicine because of the protection the government would give them against MM—something which would have been unthinkable only 10 years ago by this very conservative profession (Enthoven and Kronick, 1989; Himmelstein *et al.*, 1989).

4. US ATTEMPTS TO BREAK THE VICIOUS CIRCLE

Much litigation has already been undertaken in attempts to stop the circle both from a federal and from an individual state level. Within the past 2 years alone 44 states have proposed over 100 bills to curb MM expansion. None has so far solved the problem, some have improved the system and others have just slowed down the circle.

Measures such as the following have all been initiated as solutions and met with varying degrees of success: a national data bank on all disciplinary actions taken against physicians (Iglehart, 1987); more strict peer review control within the medical profession; lowering incentives for defensive medicine; providing reasonable statutes of limitation; controlling lawyers' contingency fees; and setting ceilings on awards, especially for pain and suffering (GAO, 1987b).

Other possible solutions still exist only as proposals: malpractice insurance rates should be set by government control boards not reinsurer companies, and the establishment of state or federal reinsurance pools would remove the pressure being exerted by the reinsurance companies.

5. MEDICAL MALPRACTICE IN DENMARK

In Denmark there is an old tradition of socialized medicine and national health insurance, where treatment is paid for by the state. Only recently have there been some very limited moves to create private 'pay-hospitals' as a sign of growing privatization in Denmark, which along with an increasing popularity of alternative healers, appears to be a response to the population's decline in belief in the established health care system.

A national economy that now demands budget cutbacks everywhere in the public sector has created hospital waiting-lists, stressed treatment conditions and dissatisfied patients and thereby a greater will among the public to ask actively for what they need and complain if it is not satisfactory. Although not nearly as dramatic as in the USA, an increasing number of claims have been filed against Danish physicians: actual negligence has been found in almost 25% of cases from the past 4 years.

For many years, claims made about medical negligence were settled in a governmental advisory board, the National Board of Health, by co-operating doctors and lawyers who, in more difficult matters (10%), consulted the Council of Forensic Medicine, consisting of medical specialists only (Rasmussen, 1988). This led to criticism of doctors' protectionism and in January 1988, a new Board was formed consisting of both professionals and laypersons—the Patient Board of Complaints. The individual patient presents his or her case to the Patient Board of Complaints, knowing that that is where the final decision is made by representatives of a wide spectrum of society.

This new system means another step is added to the bureaucratic process, but the new board serves its purpose by providing a more direct access for patients to file claims and fairer treatment of claims, since decisions are made from a commonsense perspective and not only on the basis of professional opinion.

However in order to get economic compensation for MM injuries, a patient must ask the liable party (the doctor) directly to pay for the injury through his or her liability insurance. In 1985 the medical liability insurers paid out 10 million Danish kroner (about $1.5 million) for about 200 personal injuries. If the patient disagrees with the Patient Board of Complaints' decision or the insurance company will not pay, the legal system and court are the only course left—a seldom-used and very long process in Denmark.

The punishment of the doctor found liable consists mainly of a written reprimand, 'a bloody nose', which is a very unpleasant experience in a Danish context and a scar to the honour of Danish medical professionals. If taken to court, which happens four to six times a year, the doctor may be fined or get a time-limited dismissal of licensure. The possibility of imprisonment exists but has never been used.

So what do Danes expect to get out of a claim filed, if not monetary compensation? The Patient Board of Complaints says that patients only want justice served and to know what the probable cause of malpractice was to prevent it from happening again (Patient Board of Complaints, personal communication). This serves the society as a whole, but does it help the individual patient who has already suffered? A specific detail of this discussion which has been the focus of attention recently is: What is to be done for the injured patient who did not suffer liable negligence in a legalistic sense, but has suffered 'bad luck' during extenuating medical circumstances?

In 1987, the Danish government proposed the establishment of a special Patient Insurance as already exists in Sweden and New Zealand—a 'no-fault insurance' intended to include almost all of the health care system, to compensate well defined, unavoidable complications and circumstantial accidents occurring during examinations, treatments, etc. (von Eyben, 1985).

With regard to circumstantial accidents, American lawyers state that the expression is a contradiction in terms. Negligence is a deviation from the accepted standard of care that causes damage. When a doctor takes all the necessary precautions as prescribed by the defined standard, he or she is not to be held liable for any damages. It is just a bad result. However, patients should be informed about such risks before the procedure so that they have the choice to say no.

6. COMPARISON WITH THE UK

To support the thesis of differing societal values, we shall briefly describe the phenomenon of MM in the UK, where the system appears, as in Denmark, to differ from that of the USA. In a population of approximately 55 million people, provided with (largely) free health care by the National Health Service, there were about 1000 medical malpractice claims filed in 1983, a frequency that is only a tenth of that in the USA (Miller, 1986).

Many factors, such as a different legal system, a different bureaucratic complaint system and the lower possibilities of economic compensation contribute to the much lower tendency to file suits. In British law there are no juries involved in court proceedings against malpractice—the judges find the facts, apply the law and award damages. In fact only 4% of filed claims go to court and of these, only 20% are awarded. Only recently have awards in the UK come close to the American million dollar recovery level (Miller, 1986).

Instead alternatives have emerged, in the form of three different boards handling patients' complaints about hospitals, general practitioners or administrative procedures. These boards are not only in the position of judging cases of possible negligence. It is also within their jurisdiction to propose improvement in the health care service and to recommend small ex gratia payments to patients who have suffered financial losses due to injuries.

A fourth board, whose function can be compared with state medical boards in the USA and the Council of Forensic Medicine in Denmark, acts as a disciplinary force against errant physicians. Out of 946 complaints received in 1984–1985, the Board found legal grounds for sanctions in only 21 cases. Because there is such great secrecy surrounding the Board's activities, there has been the same discussion as in Denmark and in the USA about doctor protectionism.

Finally, because of free health care and a well developed unemployment and disability compensation system, the purpose of suing and complaining is for the British patient, as for the Danish patient, usually only an attempt to receive an honest explanation, eventually an apology and an assurance that it will not happen again, leaving the economic compensation as a secondary priority.

7. SOCIAL HEALTH CARE VALUES AND PATIENT AUTONOMY

In discussing these MM phenomena, we will focus on the reasons for differences in social health care values and patient autonomy mainly in the USA and Denmark, since those in the UK appear to be so similar to Denmark. With values and economic incentives as central features and by applying a philosophy of autonomy as described in Chapter 1, we will formulate what to us seems an appropriate way of handling these signs and symptoms in health care systems.

The great difference between the MM legal response systems described is their focus on money and their connection to national economic administration. In the USA the driving force is quite clearly money, under the guise of the protection of individuals' rights. In Denmark and the UK that is less possible because justice and public protection are the primary motivation.

While American doctors work within a 'liberal' free market pricing economy with either individual patients or consumer organizations (e.g. Health Maintenance Organizations), Danish doctors must work within the socialized system with mandatory assignment directed by Danish governmental agencies and limited by fee negotiations for National Health Insurance and limits in the number of 'self-employed' general practitioners and specialists. But, more importantly, in the USA the punishment of negligent doctors is mainly motivated by legal economics. In Denmark and the UK it is driven by honour and dishonour.

Questions to be asked about the numbers of claims are: Do they really reveal the magnitude of the malpractice happenings or are they only the tip of the iceberg? And are the increases in claims a good measure of a real increase in the incidence of medical negligence or are they just revealing a greater tendency to file suits? Since a certain amount of effort, assertiveness and emotional support is needed to file a claim and since the public is becoming more conscious about its rights and possibilities in this area especially, both questions may direct a path to the answer. Furthermore a certain amount of claims should be expected every year since doctors are fallible human beings, just like the rest of society, and therefore will accidentally cause injuries occasionally in spite of every possible precaution—so-called circumstantial accidents. But is that to be accepted unconditionally by the patients? Or should the doctors be punished even though negligence cannot be found?

This leads us to ask the question: What should be defined as a 'reasonable risk' for patients receiving any prescribed treatment in terms of possible risk of damage from the treatment? 'Reasonable risk' is a concept based on the understanding that the result of a treatment is dependent on many more factors than an actual tablet or surgery, factors that cannot always be foreseen. In earlier paternalistic days, there was an inherent expectation to trust the doctor, giving him or her the benefit of the doubt if the treatment led to an unfortunate or bad result. Today, with the ever-expanding state of medical knowledge and technological development of medicine, that faith has been slowly eroded. There may have been doubts in earlier times, but they are finding expression only now in societal developmental terms. The recent explosion of the MM phenomenon as described appears to have occurred primarily because doctors do not live up to the expectations placed on them by others. Medical negligence has always existed. This is not to say that it is excused, but that it is relative.

As the economic resources available to provide services begin to fall behind technological capability, patients, regardless of their health care system, become more selective about the quality of the treatment for the price. This leads us to some further questions. What are we to do to provide justice for these accidentally injured patients? Should they just accept the injury as an unavoidable complication of that treatment? Should they be compensated economically by a mandatory patient insurance as proposed in Denmark or should they have to go to court, hoping their lawyer will be capable of proving the doctor guilty? It becomes obvious that the societal health care economic systems affect patient thinking in American and Danish models. The tolerance level of the wrongly treated Danish patient will be much higher, because he or she does not need to pay for further corrective treatments, while American patients must seek compensation, since they pay for their own retreatment. This allows the Danish doctors to define the 'reasonable risk' quite differently from their American colleagues.

This relativism is further illustrated by a discussion of physician incompetence. Removal of the wrong kidney, or failure to do house-calls when requested, are examples of obvious liable negligence. But what about the doctor who, exhausted from a tight work schedule, causes an otherwise preventable injury? Who is to blame: the doctor? the system? nobody? And who should make that judgment? In other words: Who defines the borderline between the 'reasonable risk' and the actual negligence? From what context is it defined? Is it the plaintiff's lawyer with the help of expert witnesses in court, or the state medical boards as in the USA, or is it the National Board of Health or the public as in the Patient Board of Complaints, as recently introduced in Denmark?

We can see here that the discussions of autonomy typing as described in Chapter 1 affect these phenomena and the societal selection of values created by them.

In American society the deontological perspective has a strong influence on how doctors deal with their patients in order to avoid legal suits. Through an objective or professionally distant attitude they give all possible required information about methods, results and risks and leave the subsequent decision and responsibility to the patient. Indeed the entire perspective of patient autonomy within the USA is based upon deontological ethics, with the individual in the centre, informed of all the options as a patient and yet needing to make the decision within his or her own personal economic capabilities. If one is rich, one is healthy!

Interestingly enough, the USA is also the place where the most remarkable change in concepts of autonomy has been occurring in recent years, since trends now emerge that reveal a need for a balance with social autonomy to protect both patients and doctors. We see American physicians' gestures towards a national health insurance policy in the USA as a signal for a need for a no-fault insurance policy, indicating their desire to re-establish an essentially trusting relationship with their patients, although perhaps not on a paternalistic assumption.

Here we should describe our interpretation of relativistic autonomy as an interactive model in which we believe the patient–therapist relationship is the core unit for the genesis of values. It is a model that would emphasize mutual interpersonal respect which is to be promoted at all levels of decision making, such as between the doctor and the patient or the state legislators and society as a whole. We see the interactive principle as accepting initiatives from any level of the system as long as the 'subject to subject' element of this core relationship promotes trust and mutual respect, as in the 19th century doctor–patient relationship before higher technologies and third-party pressures became complicating factors. This is not to say that the paternalism of that era is desirable today. But the mutual respect and interactive nature of the relationship is desirable and based on equality of social standing of doctor and patient roles.

In the social autonomy paradigm as advanced in Chapter 1, we see no 'person object' forming the basis of caring. It is harder to care about the state or a bureaucratic organization (e.g. WHO) with all its inevitable complexities, standardizations and physical distance. And who decides on what values to support weaker elements in society? Who determines these persons' points of view? We fear that state paternalism will set goals and values for patients and that it could have less personal meaning for them than even the older deontological paternalism of the 19th century.

We believe the social autonomy model is the perspective in Denmark and the UK, where the state has taken the responsibility of providing sufficient health care to every member of its society, including the maltreated, thus diminishing the economic incentive to sue and ask for compensation and the need for doctors to protect themselves from their patients. A consequence of this type of autonomy, which protects individual rights to a lesser degree, is that it expresses, through political decisions, definitive solutions to problems occurring within its society, thereby placing the state in the authoritative expert role—a role that has in recent history been denied to the medical profession more and more by both the public and the state. Authority still exists, only now at a higher, less definable and much less personable level.

Questions are raised: Is an authority needed as the ultimate decision maker? How is social autonomy to be operated for patients in their own context? Another example beyond the MM issue is the recent debate in Denmark of hip versus heart operations. In a time when there are limited National Health Insurance funds, the Danes are faced with the difficult choice between improvement of the quality of life of a greater number of people through hip replacements and the option of life or death for a smaller number through more expensive heart transplantations. It is a discussion that occurs less frequently in the USA given the deontological perspective, where patients options and restrictions are set by their own socioeconomic capacity. It is here more a question of whether the patient is rich or insured and gets a new heart, or poor, uneducated and less resourceful and does not get a transplant.

The philosophy of autonomies described in Chapter 1 can also be interpreted as different perceptions of social values as basic principles working at different levels within any health care system. In administering national health care systems today, including managing the problem of MM, the social autonomy principle as we interpret it is apparent. Politicians (more in Denmark than in the USA) make laws to deal with the economically disadvantaged, thereby either trying to provide more equal health care possibilities or creating restrictions for everyone. Whereas, at the level of daily routine in hospitals and offices, the deontological and relativistic principles mingle with each other with each patient the doctor meets, dependent on the personalities of the patient and the doctor. In MM court cases, American lawyers tend to enforce the deontological component of patient autonomy by asking definitive answers to complex problems on behalf of patients. But confusingly, they also express the relativistic point of view, defining the plaintiff's damaged quality of life that goes beyond physical damage and thus demand monetary compensation for 'pain and suffering'.

But no matter which economic system or what type or level of autonomy can be applied, we see a degeneration of the doctor–patient relationship, probably the most serious problem related to the MM phenomenon, since the phenomenon interferes with the essential basic trust within this relationship and reflects its decline. There is a decline in not only the old paternalistic view of the doctor, wherever it may still exist, but also in the natural belief in an approachable, reliable and competent doctor, thus creating feelings of insecurity and powerlessness for patients in any contact with the health care system. This loss in patients' confidence is signalled by the increasing number of law suits and has led to a further devaluation of the principle of equality of access to treatment in the USA, as exemplified by some doctors refusing to treat some Medicare patients who might sue them.

In Denmark, this lack of confidence and patient dissatisfaction has led to an increasing interest and attention to alternative treatment forms, such as chinesiology and 'healing'—unfortunately, often without the natural scepticism inherent in this well informed society. But why? Though varied in their offers and philosophies of treatment, the alternative therapists have one thing in common: the extra time they give and the interest they show the individual patient and his or her problems in the context of his or her daily life. Thus, the decline in patient confidence signals a demand among patients for rights, knowledge and justice. It may stimulate patient assertiveness, but just how are these demands to be fulfilled? Which model of autonomy of action is preferable to serve the larger needs of the society and the individual at the same time?

The examples above point to the need for support of the interpersonal interaction between doctor and patient, since it is easier to know the neighbourhood doctor than the state. But the state should create the grounds for this relationship—a type of autonomy we will call an interactive version of relativistic autonomy with socially autonomous reinforcement of the doctor–patient relationship. Both the doctor and the patient must feel responsible for their actions in this essential relationship.

8. CONCLUSION

From this description it appears that the MM phenomenon is less developed in Denmark and the UK than in the USA, because Danish and British cultures and health care systems do not have the same emphasis on values about private enterprise and individual rights as there is in the USA. In the USA, MM is largely a business phenomenon, catalysed by the legal profession in which complacency of medical state boards about incompetent members has led to the punishment of the profession as a whole. In all three nations the phenomenon of MM is promoted and reinforced by societal changes that question the physicians as the ultimate medical authority (paternalism) in the context of patient values. This is not necessarily wrong, but it has perhaps led to other serious problems.

There is a need to define the problem, of which the symptoms are the explosive and complex MM phenomenon. To us it seems obvious that the very centre of this situation is in fact the site of a solution: the doctor–patient relationship. By recognizing that this does provide a solution, one sees the importance of putting major effort into preserving the good qualities of this relationship since, through that effort, so many misunderstandings could be prevented and huge personal and physical injuries might never occur. Distress and anger could be avoided and money and time could be saved. By highlighting this aspect of the health care system, it is emphasized that the responsibility for the public's health rests mainly with each individual, but that this must be supported by the respected, concerned engagement of their doctor—a concept of patient autonomy at a basic level of mutual interest and health caring.

By supporting and strengthening the interactive quality of the doctor–patient relating by whatever means available and striving for mutual respect and interpersonal confidence, the MM problem would dissolve in a wider societal context. To work from here one must know that it is a long-term objective to change what is happening, since it involves altering attitudes, cultural values and human nature. Thus it becomes the responsibility of both the individual person and society as a whole to make changes in medical practice more complete and acceptable.

We suggest that neither the rights of the individual patient at the expense of the whole society nor the rights of the whole society versus individual rights should be the focus of MM proceedings as evidenced in the American, Danish and British models presented. Rather, government and medical professional leaders (for example, WHO) should strive to provide new incentives for improving the doctor–patient relationship, while also setting concrete realistic guidelines for what constitutes 'reasonable risk' in the treatment of patients, starting with the education of physicians. The doctor should be a 'patient advocate' who in his or her promotion of the patient's treatment creates an atmosphere of security and trust through an attitude that may sometimes be objective, sometimes concerned, but never uncritical in giving information, taking into account the specific physical and emotional needs of the individual patient. The doctor also needs security and trust, which means that the economic incentives for 'lottery syndrome' law suits for circumstantial accidents must abate. This poses mutually identifiable needs for both these roles within the relationship.

Such a perspective might best be promoted through legislation of economic or structural incentives within the health care system that will make it easier for patients to feel more secure with doctors and vice versa. Education and information at all levels for both public and professionals are important, and the following should be emphasized:

1. Positive values like interpersonal involvement, genuine concern and confidence and trust—putting the value of 'care' back into the term 'health care'—encouraging doctors to care about their patients as persons and not only as diseases or possible law suit risks.
2. Improvement in communication within the doctor–patient relationship so that both parties become clear about each other's expectations. This could be information about a treatment and its consequent risks or about personal symptoms, problems or insecurity related to treatment. Interpersonal communication skills should be actively taught and exercised in medical education.
3. Education of the public to have realistic expectations about physicians (they are human and not infallible), medical care (what is possible and what is not), the law (what is the patient's right) and the doctor–patient relationship. The goal is to make patients more responsible for the treatment they get because they want it, not because the doctor wants it, making them more self-aware, so that they know what the problem is and then what to ask for. Patient information must be presented accurately and in written form wherever possible.

   Education must be directed toward the public in general and the patients and their families/surroundings in particular. With the increasing number of chronically ill individuals, it is important that the family understands what is happening so as to prevent subsequent misunderstandings with physicians and know how the family can best support these patients.

These suggestions can enhance the values of caring and stimulate interpersonal involvement, which should be the building blocks of all health care systems, regardless of the political or economic system.

REFERENCES

Appleby, C. R. (1987) St Paul Co seeks rate hikes. *Health Week*, September 28, 15–16.

Coleman, B. (1989) States act against unfit docs. *AARP News Bulletin* **1**, 1.

Danzon, P. M. (1984) Testimony presented to the Committee on Labor and Human Resources, US Senate. July 10.

Enthoven, A. and Kronick, R. (1989) A consumer-choice health plan for the 1990s. *New England Journal of Medicine* **1**, 29–37, **2**, 94–101.

GAO (1986) *Medical Malpractice: No agreement on the Problems or Solutions*. US government report GAO/HRD-86–50.

GAO (1987a) *Medical Malpractice: Characteristics of Claims Closed in 1984*. US government report GAO/HRD-87–55.

GAO (1987b) *Medical Malpractice: A Framework for Action*. US government report GAO/HRD-87–73.

Himmelstein, D. U. *et al.* (1989) A national health program for the United States. *New England Journal of Medicine* **2**, 102–7.

Huttmann, B. (1981) *The Patient's Advocate*. Viking Press, New York.

Iglehart, J. K. (1987) Congress moves to bolster peer review: the Health Care Quality Improvement Act of 1986. *New England Journal of Medicine* **316**, 960–4.

Mayer, D. (1987) AAFP shops for insurers. *Health Week*, September 28, 15.

Miller, F. H. (1986) Medical malpractice litigation: do the British have a better remedy? *American Journal of Law and Medicine* **11**, 433–63.

Rasmussen, J. (1988) *Det Iatrogene Ansvar—om Lægers Ansvar, (The Iatrogenic Responsibility—about Doctors' Responsibility)*. FADL's Forlag, Denmark.

Relman, A. (1987) Practicing medicine in the new business climate. *New England Journal of Medicine* **316**, 1150–4.

Sabiston, D. C. (1985) Professional liability in the 1980s: problems and solutions. *Bulletin of the American College of Surgeons* **70**, 6–11.

von Eyben, B. (1985) *Lægeansvar fra Medicinsk Etik* (*Doctors' responsibility from Ethics of Medicine*). FADL's Forlag, Denmark, pp. 216–40.

Winkenweider, W. and Ball, J. R. (1988) Transformation of American health care; the role of the medical profession. *New England Journal of Medicine* **318**, 317–19.

13

Resource Allocation in Health Care: The Role of the Courts

Kenneth McK. Norrie, LLB, DLP, PhD

1. INTRODUCTION

Resource allocation in health care is all about making decisions. These decisions may be general policy matters—whether to open a hospital here, or to close an organ transplantation unit there—or they may involve choices between individuals—whether to send Mr Roe home from hospital because it is decided that Mr Smith needs the bed—or they may involve choices of treatment for individuals—whether Mrs Brown's condition should be treated by expensive surgery or by cheaper drug therapy. All such decisions, whether taken by the state or a local health administrative unit or an individual doctor, will at the end of the day affect individual patients, who are relying on the medical profession to cure them of some ill, or to alleviate some physical or mental condition.

However, most patients realise that they cannot get everything they may want, either from the state or from the medical profession. Resources are finite and must be spread amongst those who have valid calls upon them, and someone must therefore decide what calls are valid and how the resource allocation is to be made. Few patients would deny that need, and demand as an absolute right that these decisions should always be made in their own favour. The vast majority of patients will however expect and insist upon the decisions being made in a fair and reasonable manner. Every individual who makes a call upon the resources allocated by society to health care will expect to be given fair consideration, equal to that given to his or her neighbour. And that expectation of equal treatment is not only deep-rooted into our notions of democracy and justice but is also reflected in the western legal tradition.

Changing Values in Medical and Health Care Decision Making
Edited by U. J. Jensen and G. Mooney

It sometimes happens however that an individual is dissatisfied with the way the medical profession has treated him or her. If a resource allocation decision has been made which is detrimental to a particular individual, that individual may be tempted to believe that he or she has been treated unjustly, or has not been given the same consideration as that received by other patients. In the face of such dissatisfaction it is understandable that a patient may turn to the law, which *purports* to provide justice and *professes* to treat everyone equally. When this happens, the values relevant to the individual come into conflict with the values adopted by the decision maker—and it is for the court to resolve such a conflict. But in doing so the court will inevitably utilise its own values, which may be very different to the values in conflict, since they have evolved in a different way and in response to different pressures. Indeed the court's values exist at a different level of abstraction from those in conflict before it.

Litigation is in its fundament a consequence of a conflict of values; and over the past decade or so there has been in many countries in Europe and North America a vast increase in litigation against the medical profession. But it is likely that this has come about not through any change in the relative values of either doctor or patient, but rather through a change in attitude of patients towards doctors. No longer are doctors perceived as the people who always know best, the people who cannot be criticised; for people, in all aspects of life, are becoming more aware of their rights and are more willing to complain when they seem to be threatened. This can only be a good thing, for it will encourage the medical profession to think about the consequences of its actions, and to rationalise and justify, rather than simply accept, the values by which it lives and works. No less importantly, the move from paternalism to autonomy described in Chapter 1 of this book is reflected in changed attitudes in the law. Legal standards of care expected of doctors used to follow the paternalistic model of medicine; now they tend to reflect autonomy, regarding that as fundamental to personal liberty, and encouraging, in the process, a greater readiness to challenge medical providers and decision makers.

Litigation has recently begun to involve arguments about resource allocation. The law in most countries had nothing to say on this matter before such litigation was commenced: it had effectively no precise values by which to judge such disputes. This chapter will therefore examine more the evolving than the changing of values. The real change (which can be seen in all areas of litigation) is in the individual's increased willingness to challenge governmental or quasi-governmental decisions.

This chapter will examine the various bases available in common law jurisdictions to patients seeking to influence resource allocation decisions, and also how some courts, particularly those in the UK, have dealt with patients coming to them to ask the court to become involved in resource allocation decisions. (Though the examples are mostly British, the legal principles they illustrate are applicable far more generally.) After that will be identified a few of the values that the courts have evolved in the determination of whether they ought to become involved in the decision making process of resource allocation in health care. Such values are not applicable to only one or a few legal systems, but may assist any country's courts faced with the same problems.

2. THE BASES OF ACTIONABILITY

There are three major bases upon which an aggrieved individual can go to a court in a common law country (i.e. a country following the Anglo-American legal tradition) challenging a health care decision, or asking for a resource allocation decision to be made in a particular way:

1. Breach of statutory duty.
2. Judicial review.
3. Negligence.

2.1. Breach of statutory duty

If legislation imposes a duty on any person to act in a certain way, and that person does not so act, then that person may be taken to court by any other person affected by that failure to act. If the court accepts that there has been a failure to perform a duty, then it can order the person to fulfil his or her statutory duty, and it would be contempt of court for him or her then to fail to do so (which could lead to a fine or even imprisonment). The court can also make a monetary award of damages against the person who breaches his or her statutory duty, if that breach causes loss, injury or damage. An Act of Parliament can impose duties on anyone, and this includes the Government itself. This can be illustrated by the English case of *Meade* v. *London Borough Council of Haringey* (1979). Under the Education Act 1944 the British Secretary of State for Education has a duty to provide schools and educational services for all children in England and Wales under a certain age. In 1978, due to strike action by school-workers, London schools were closed, and the Secretary of State could not therefore provide education during the currency of the strike. He had no power to order an end to the strike: in other words, there was nothing he could do about his own failure to fulfil his statutory duty to provide educational services. But when he was taken to court by an aggrieved parent, the court found in favour of the parent and granted a decree ordering him to fulfil his statutory duty to provide school services. Damages were also awarded.

This case is important for two reasons. First, it shows that Government decisions in the UK are open to challenge in the courts. And secondly, it shows that the Government cannot rely on the defence that there is nothing it can do about the situation, or that the breach of duty occurred because of events or circumstances outside its control. If Parliament has imposed a duty, said the court, the Government must carry it out.

The analogy between education services and health services is strong, for many governments also have statutory duties to provide health care. The decision in *Meade* would seem to suggest that the British Government could not claim lack of resources as a defence to its failure to provide a particular medical service, and that a patient who did not receive the medical treatment he or she either wanted or needed could therefore sue the government. But in fact this has not been the approach adopted by the British courts, and different considerations have been held relevant in the medical situation from those relevant in education.

The British Government certainly has a number of obligations imposed upon it by the statutes that set up the British National Health Service. The current legislation is the National Health Service Act 1977 and the National Health Service (Scotland) Act 1978. Under these Acts of Parliament the relevant Government minister has a duty: 'to provide . . . to such extent as he considers necessary to meet all reasonable requirements: (a) hospital accommodation . . . (c) medical, dental, nursing and ambulance services . . . (f) such other services as are required for the diagnosis and treatment of illness'.

In 1980, the British Government was taken to court on an allegation that it had breached this statutory duty. This was in the case of *Regina* v. *Secretary of State for Social Services, ex parte Hincks & Ors* (1980), and it reached the Court of Appeal, which was presided over by Lord Denning, the same judge as had presided in the previous education case of *Meade*.

The *Hincks* case was raised by four patients who had waited for a number of years to be given hip replacements. They claimed that their operations were being postponed for an unreasonably long time, because of the decision of the Secretary of State not to build a new wing of a hospital on the grounds of cost. They argued that the resources issue was irrelevant and that lack of resources provided no defence: if Parliament imposed a duty to provide medical facilities, the Government must provide these facilities, and could not plead lack of cash. It sounded very like the education case. But this time the case failed. The court held that the Government was not guilty of a breach of statutory duty because the words of the statute gave the Secretary of State a wide discretion as to the allocation of scarce resources. The Act imposes a duty on the Secretary of State to provide medical services 'to such extent as *he* considers necessary to meet all reasonable requirements'. This form of words implies that a discretion is given to the Secretary of State to make decisions in the way that he considers appropriate. The court pointed out that the Secretary of State's responsibility was to the whole of the National Health Service and not to any single hospital or any single patient. Lord Denning held that there had to be implied into the obligation to provide health services a qualification limiting the duty to 'within the resources available'. He continued as follows:

> It cannot be supposed that the Secretary of State has to provide all the latest equipment. . . . It cannot be supposed that the Secretary of State has to provide all the kidney machines which are asked for, or for all the new developments such as heart transplants in every case where people would benefit from them. It cannot be supposed that the Secretary of State has a duty to provide everything that is asked for in the changed circumstances which have come about. That includes the numerous pills that people take nowadays: it cannot be said that he has to provide all these free for everybody.

It would follow that the Secretary of State would be liable only when he is shown to have committed a positive abuse of his powers, such as for example spending money allocated to health care on a political propaganda campaign designed, say, to encourage people to turn to private medicine. But a mere failure to provide services would not result in liability (unless that itself amounted to such an abuse).

A similar decision was reached in the Scottish case of *Bonthrone* v. *Secretary of State for Scotland* (1987), in which a patient had challenged the Government's campaign to encourage the vaccination of children against whooping cough. The Scottish court held that the decision to spend money on such a campaign was one that the Government had the power to make, under the discretion given by the National Health Service (Scotland) Act 1978, and therefore that decision could not be challenged, either by anyone who thought the money should be spent elsewhere, or by a person who was allegedly injured as a result of the campaign (i.e. as a result of accepting vaccination).

2.2. Judicial review

The second legal basis of an action before the courts open to patients complaining about decisions is judicial review of administrative action. Very basically, if any public body makes a decision that will affect other people, then the affected person may challenge the decision on the ground that it was unreasonable and ought therefore to be overturned. There are two significant questions that must be asked in relation to judicial review. First, is the body making the decision a 'public' body? For it is only decisions containing a public element (i.e. that affect the public) that can be challenged by way of judicial review. Secondly, if the first question is answered affirmatively, is the decision 'unreasonable' in the legal sense of that word?

A local health authority or public hospital (i.e. one to which members of the public have access, whether for payment or not) are both clearly public bodies, and so a health authority or a hospital administration that decides to divert its resources in a particular direction may potentially have that decision challenged. On the other hand, it is much more difficult to bring decisions by individual health care workers within the scope of 'public' for the purposes of judicial review. In the English case of *Regina* v. *Ethical Committee of St Mary's Hospital, ex parte Harriott* (1988), a consultant obstetrician had refused to accept a woman onto her in vitro fertilisation programme within the National Health Service. The woman sought judicial review against the obstetrician and the hospital ethical committee that had affirmed the obstetrician's decision. The judge held that some of the Committee's decisions might in certain (unspecified) cases be open to judicial review, but in relation to the obstetrician he avoided the issue of whether her decision was public by holding that the decision was clearly reasonable and therefore could not be challenged whether or not it was public. The availability of judicial review over decisions of individual doctors is therefore in some doubt in English law.

It is interesting to compare this case with the Canadian decision in *Re Medhurst & Medhurst* et al. (1984). In Canadian law [until the Supreme Court decision in *Morgentaler, Smoling & Scott* v. *The Queen* (1988)] abortion was legal only when a hospital therapeutic abortion committee decided that the statutory conditions for abortion had been fulfilled. In *Medhurst* it was decided that such a committee, being a statutory creation established to perform public functions, was clearly a public body and therefore open to judicial review.

From these cases we can deduce that in legal systems allowing for judicial review of administrative action it is likely that an individual doctor's decisions concerning the treatment of individual patients are matters purely private to doctor and patient (and therefore not open to judicial review). On the other hand the decisions of health authorities, government officials, and quasi-governmental bodies are clearly public (and therefore open to judicial review). But doctors, or ethical committees, often make decisions about individuals that have public effects, because they are in essence policy decisions (e.g. that individuals within a certain category will not be treated or will be treated a certain way). These are, it is suggested, sufficiently public decisions to be open to judicial review.

Once it has been established that the decision is a 'public' one, the applicant must then go on to prove that it is legally unreasonable, and ought therefore to be overturned. An unreasonable decision in law is one that is based on irrelevant considerations, or one that is so absurd that no sensible person would ever have made it, or one that is made in bad faith [*Associated Provincial Picture Houses Ltd.* v. *Wednesbury Corporation* (1948)]. This is a very strict test: the applicant must show not only that the decision would be considered unreasonable by the court, but also that the decision is such that no reasonable decision maker would have come to it. In the *Harriott* case mentioned above, the decision to refuse in vitro fertilisation treatment to a woman who had a criminal record in prostitution and brothel keeping was considered not to be unreasonable in this sense because it was not one that no reasonable decision maker would have come to.

In relation to resource allocation, this can be illustrated by two very similar cases from the English Court of Appeal. In *Regina* v. *Secretary of State for Social Services, ex parte Walker* (1987) a mother raised an action against the Birmingham Health Authority on behalf of her baby son, who required an operation on a valve in his heart. The operation had been postponed a number of times due to nursing shortages, and the mother claimed that it was unreasonable for the Health Authority to have failed to train enough specialist nurses. The Court of Appeal refused the application. Sir John Donaldson said this:

> It is not for this court, or indeed for any court, to substitute its own judgment for the judgment of those who are responsible for the allocation of resources.

But interestingly and importantly, the Court of Appeal did emphasise that it would be open to the courts to overturn a resource allocation decision if it had been made in an unreasonable fashion, or had unreasonable consequences. 'The jurisdiction does exist', said the court, asserting that it does indeed have the ultimate right to overturn a particular resource allocation decision, though it did not do so in this particular case.

Shortly afterwards an identical case again reached the Court of Appeal. This was *Regina* v. *Central Birmingham Health Authority, ex parte Collier* (1988), and the only extra element in this case was that there seemed to be much more of an emergency facing the baby boy here, in the sense that he was much nearer death than was the Walker baby. But the same decision was reached by the court as in the previous case. Lord Justice Stephen Brown in *Collier* said:

> The courts of this country cannot arrange the lists in the hospitals, and, if there is no evidence that they are not being arranged properly due to some unreasonableness . . . the courts cannot, and should not, be asked to intervene.

Lord Justice Ralph Gibson said that the courts 'have no role of general investigator of social policy or of allocation of resources'. But again, it was emphasised that a health authority's decision on resource allocation can be challenged, though such a challenge will only be successful if the decision can be shown to have been made unreasonably, in the *Wednesbury* sense described above.

Clearly each case will be looked at on its own merits, and it is difficult to predict the sort of decisions that the court will consider unreasonable. The cases discussed above do however suggest that it would only be in highly exceptional circumstances that a legal challenge to a resource allocation decision will be sustained. Clearly a decision will not be considered to have been made unreasonably if it takes into account the total resources available to the decision maker, because the court recognises that reasonable decision makers invariably are governed by the resources at their disposal. A decision is not therefore unreasonable just because it favours one patient over another. A decision will be unreasonable in law only when it is such that no rational decision maker would have made it had he or she borne in mind all the relevant facts of the particular case. This is a very difficult test to satisfy, and so long as the decision maker is careful and rational, and bears in mind only relevant considerations, then it is unlikely that his, her or its decision will be overturned in a court of law.

2.3. Negligence

The third basis of claim available in the Anglo-American legal systems would be for the patient to allege that the decision maker has acted negligently. In law negligence is an unreasonable failure to prevent injury in circumstances in which one ought reasonably to have foreseen one's actions would cause injury. Negligence against a doctor is notoriously difficult to prove in most legal systems. The claimant must establish three things: unreasonable behaviour, loss injury or damage, and a causal connexion between the two. Unreasonableness is defined very similarly to its definition for the purposes of judicial review. The *locus classicus* in the UK is the following statement of Lord President Clyde in the Scottish case of *Hunter* v. *Hanley* (1955), which may be taken as representing the test in other jurisdictions also:

> The true test for establishing negligence . . . on the part of a doctor is whether he has been proved to be guilty of such failure as no doctor of ordinary skill would be guilty of if acting with ordinary care.

But even when liability for negligence can be established, this is not a very helpful action from the decision maker's point of view. It is always a retrospective action, in the sense that it can only deal with injuries already suffered, and it gives very little guidance as to how future decision makers should act. Some guidance can however be gleaned from how the law treats other decision makers in different circumstances.

The law generally does not tolerate people making decisions on the basis of values that do not coincide with the court's own. This can be seen from two 19th century cases in which life or death decisions had to be made. Both involved shipwrecks with survivors stranded in lifeboats. In the first, *US* v. *Holmes* (1841), a ship sank and a number of people clambered onto a lifeboat. There were too many people and the lifeboat would certainly sink, drowning everyone. A ship's officer then decided who to throw overboard, and Holmes carried out the instructions: so killing those whom he threw into the water, but saving a larger number. Holmes was convicted of manslaughter, and the appeal court upheld his conviction. The judges indicated that the ship's officer had no authority or right to make the decisions himself: rather, the court held, he should have organised some sort of lottery (which would effectively put the matter in the hands of fate, or an all-powerful god). In a similar English case, *Regina* v. *Dudley and Stephens* (1884), two men and a cabin boy found themselves adrift in a lifeboat with no food. The two men killed and ate the cabin boy after 20 days of starvation. Again, the court held them rightly convicted of manslaughter. The English court said that they should have done nothing (even though the most likely outcome of that was death for all three).

How does this help decision makers in health care? It would seem to suggest that they must leave the matter to fate (or the deity), or must make no decision. They could do both by adopting a 'first come, first served' approach, and give all their time and resources to the patient who presents for treatment chronologically before any other patient. This leaves it to fate to determine who comes first, and avoids the doctor making decisions on the basis of his or her own values. Yet, even if this approach were morally justifiable (which, it is suggested, it is not as it is no more than an abrogation of one's duty to uncontrolled fortuitousness), it is not as easy of application as it might appear. When does a person first present for a 'first come, first served' approach? A patient with a bad kidney may go for years before it deteriorates sufficiently to require dialysis. Is he in front of the queue before people who suddenly suffer acute kidney failure? That decision has to be made, so once again it is left to the individual doctor. However, so long as the decision satisfies the court's definition of reasonableness, it will be unchallengeable.

It is often said that different considerations are to be taken into account once the doctor has decided to treat a patient, and that once treatment is commenced, it should not be withdrawn while the patient still needs it. In other words, a doctor cannot stop one person's treatment to give it to another when a more needy (in the doctor's view) patient presents for treatment. Though this may be considered by some to be ethically sound, there is certainly no legal rule to this effect, and the courts are unlikely to criticise a decision to terminate treatment unless that decision is as unreasonable as the decision not to provide treatment in the first place. Oxford Health Authority came in for much criticism in the British press in 1985 (see Brahams, 1985). A 42-year-old man was put on haemodialysis to save his life. He responded badly to the treatment, though in an emotional rather than a physical sense. He was a tramp, mentally immature, homeless, unemployed, dirty, abusive, and profoundly ungrateful for his treatment. The health authority terminated his treatment by reallocating his dialysis place to a clean, employed, courteous man who later became in need of the treatment in order to save his life.

It is unlikely that the court would have overturned that decision had it been legally challenged. The courts do recognise and accept that considerations other than purely medical ones are relevant, and, while there are not sufficient resources for all, then a decision will not be considered to have been made unreasonably or negligently just because an inevitable consequence of it is the death of an individual patient.

3. VALUES RELEVANT TO THE COURT

So what then is the true role of the courts in resource allocation in health care? And what should it be? In the cases discussed above, the courts have proved themselves extremely reluctant to become at all involved in the decision making process. But the courts are not completely closed. It is clear from the cases mentioned above that if the patient can show that a decision has been wholly unreasonable, in the sense already discussed, then that decision can be overturned, and damages can be awarded to anyone injured by the decision.

That is the extent of the role that the courts, certainly in the UK, are willing to take in decision making in resource allocation. It must be asked whether it is right and sensible of them to have limited themselves in this way, or whether they—or any other country's courts—ought to adopt a much more active role in decision making. There are a number of arguments on both sides that courts in any jurisdiction might consider relevant.

3.1. Advantages of the court action

The availability of the court action brings certain advantages. In the first place, courts can force treatment to be given that would not otherwise be given, and so save lives. In the *Walker* and *Collier* cases, even though the patients lost their cases, the very fact of taking the matters to court publicised the shortages of specialist nursing and the health authority felt obliged to carry out the operations soon afterwards. (The baby Walker died shortly after his operation.) Of course the resources have to come from somewhere, but it might be argued that the courts can make a more dispassionate judgment on this matter than the health authorities or hospitals.

In the second place, and more importantly, courts are open and public and accountable for their decisions. Too often decisions made by health authorities are made secretly and it is not known on what values they based their decisions. They may have used the wrong values, but no one can tell because the process normally is secret, or, as the decision makers might put it, confidential.

In the third place, the court system provides a right of appeal that would not exist otherwise. There is a lot to be said for giving a right of appeal to anyone against any form of decision that could lead to that person's death. If a hospital has one place on a dialysis machine, and two patients need the place to live, the decision to give it to one will result in the death of the other. But the condemned person has no appeal from such a decision. This sits uneasily with western notions of due process of law, protected in for example, the European Convention on Human Rights, the US Constitution, and the Canadian Charter on Rights and Freedoms.

In the fourth place, the courts can impose national standards of decision making, and ensure that the same values are adopted throughout the country. At the moment in the UK each area health authority and local health board makes its own decisions based upon the criteria it considers relevant, which may be very different from the criteria adopted in other areas. Ability to pay, homelessness, employability and cleanliness *may* be relevant criteria to affect the health care decision, but none is self-evidently so, and none is unanimously accepted or rejected across the country. The courts can lay down single standards, to be followed by all. There is no room in the law for local values, and there should be none in health care provision either: for health ought to be regarded as an asset equally valuable to everyone wherever they live, and no matter their age, occupation, religion, sex, or whatever. One of the greatest values recognised by the law is equality of treatment for everyone within each legal system's jurisdiction, and this is a value the law will—and ought to—continue to impose.

3.2. Disadvantages of the court action

But there are strong counter-arguments to all of the above, reflecting greater values recognised by the law. First, if the courts did adopt a much more active role in health care decision making, they would undoubtedly be swamped with applications by people feeling that they are not receiving correct treatment. Any patient with a grievance, or on a waiting list for any form of treatment, whether therapeutic or elective, would be tempted to go to court. The hospital waiting lists would be turned into court waiting lists, and no one would be any better off (except possibly the lawyers).

Secondly, it is not for the courts, or for doctors, or economists, or philosophers (as is pointed out in Chapter 1 of this book), to make policy decisions on the allocation of national resources. Rather it is for our elected representatives in Parliament. The courts cannot determine whether elective treatment such as family planning and birth control is more important to the national good than is, say, the heart transplantation programme. These national decisions of social policy are not for the courts to make. It is for Parliament, no one else.

Thirdly, with more individual decisions, the courts really do not have the specialist knowledge required to determine issues that revolve around medical need. A choice between one drug, say, rather than another is a medical decision, not a legal one. Medical decisions concerning individuals' treatment are nearly always made on the basis of medical need, and it would be cumbersome and impracticable to have to prove that need to the legal and non-medical minds that preside in most courts of law.

Fourthly, and most significantly, decision making in health care would be reduced to its worst possible basis—the likelihood of court action if a decision is not made to favour a particular individual. This is not—and must never be allowed to become—a 'value' in the decision making process. At the moment most resource allocation decisions are made on the basis of medical priorities, or economic priorities, or political priorities, or philosophical priorities, or a combination of these things. All have their advantages and all may be justified on their own terms. What would have no justification at all however would be to make decisions to favour patients on the basis of which patient is most likely to go to court, or who is most likely to make a fuss in public about an adverse decision. The Walker and Collier babies received their operations to prevent any further adverse criticism in the British press, but the resources were taken from other areas where there was no such criticism. That consideration has nothing whatsoever to do with health and is based on wholly irrelevant factors, and any decision based upon it is therefore in itself unreasonable. The result of the courts taking an active role in medical decision making would be that Mrs Jones would be given her hip replacement before Mr Doe because Mrs Jones criticises and challenges and complains, while Mr Doe is timid and quiet and would not think of criticising his doctor. Resources would be given to infertility research rather than to geriatric care because the pressure group for infertile patients is far stronger and more vociferous than the geriatric lobby. The result of the courts taking a more active role in the decision making process is that those with the loudest voices would benefit most.

4. CONCLUSION

It is clear that, if they were to take an active role, the courts could affect the relative weights to be given to the values adopted by the health care professions in their resource allocation decisions, and in this way change these values themselves. However the courts have been content to adopt a more *reactive* approach, reflecting the changing values of society itself, through the concept of reasonableness. The courts use this concept to reflect current ideas of worth, morality, fairness and rationality, and its inherent amorphousness allows the courts to adjust it when it perceives that society's values have changed. In most other areas the courts in any country do not hesitate to apply their own values to disputes before them, thus leading the changes, rather than reacting to them; but the dangers mentioned above of the courts attempting to do this in relation to resource allocation decisions are both real and obvious, and must not be under-rated. The British courts are clearly aware of these dangers, and have resisted the temptation to take on an active rather than a reactive role in changing values. For all the reasons given above, it is suggested that this is as it should be.

REFERENCES

Associated Provincial Picture Houses Ltd. v. *Wednesbury Corporation* [1948] K.B. 230.
Bonthrone v. *Secretary of State for Scotland* 1987 SLT 34.
Brahams (1985) A doctor's justification for withdrawing treatment. *New Law Journal*, **48**, 135.
Hunter v. *Hanley* 1955 SC 200.
Meade v. *London Borough Council of Haringey* [1979] 2 All ER 1016.
Morgentaler, Smoling and Scott v. *The Queen* [1988] 44 DLR (4th) 385.
R. v. *Central Birmingham Health Authority, ex parte Collier* (unreported) 6th January 1988, Court of Appeal.
R. v. *Dudley and Stephens* (1884) 14 QBD 273.
R. v. *Ethical Committee of St Mary's Hospital, ex parte Harriott* (1988) Fam. Law 165.
R. v. *Secretary of State for Social Services, ex parte Hincks & Ors* (unreported) 18th March 1980, Court of Appeal.
R. v. *Secretary of State for Social Services, ex parte Walker* (unreported) 26th November 1987, Court of Appeal.
Re Medhurst and Medhurst et al. (1984) 7 DLR (4th) 335.
US v. *Holmes* (1841) 26 Fed. Cas. 360.

14

Changing Values and Changing Policy

Gavin Mooney, MA and Uffe Juul Jensen, PhD

In this final chapter we do not wish to try to summarise what has gone before or to try to bring all the previous chapters together in some common frame of reference. Rather we would like to concentrate on certain aspects of the central issue addressed in this book in all chapters, that is the question of changing values in medicine and health care. We have chosen to do this in the context of policy and to choose what we see as certain key but not all-embracing aspects, which have in fact been at least touched on in the preceding pages. These are the links between the values of medicine and the values of health care and the question of the changing role and values underlying equity.

It can be argued that there has always been a tension between many of the values underlying medicine and those on which health care policy are based. It seems unlikely however that these tensions have ever been as great as they are today. Medicine, or at least its dominant clinical component, remains fixed, in training and in outlook in practice, in a world where individual values are paramount. Health care as essentially a social institution cannot be other than based on social values. Yet it is only in comparatively recent years that anything approximating to a sense of conflict has arisen between these different sets of values and indeed the (in principle) separable institutions of medicine and health care.

The reasons for change here are several. That which has perhaps received most attention is that associated with the economic and financial environment surrounding health care at present and indeed has done since the halcyon economic growth days of the 1960s. The slowing in the rate of growth of real resources in the health sector, and in some countries an actual fall, has resulted in the realisation in both medical and non-medical quarters

Changing Values in Medical and Health Care Decision Making
Edited by U. J. Jensen and G. Mooney

of the need for change in the values underlying both medicine and health care.

It is quite inconceivable that such an eminent medical personage as Hoffenberg, the President of the Royal College of Physicians in the UK, would have been writing in the 1960s, as he has recently in the 1980s, about the justifiable limits to clinical freedom that economic constraints impose (Hoffenberg, 1987). It is not a wholly new phenomenon and has a pedigree stretching back to Archie Cochrane (1972) in the early 1970s in his concerns with both effectiveness and efficiency in medical practice. These ideas have been taken up in turn by Jennett (1983) in his expressed concerns with the failures of the medical profession to assess new technologies properly before implementing them. It is the approaching respectability of the ideas of Hoffenberg that is the major shift here. There is no longer the same sense of outrage among the profession that such views are expressed by their own members. Not that they are common views even today. The old guard remain and in high positions. Thus Gøtrik, the President of the Danish Medical Association, was claiming as recently as 1987 that since it was doctors who were in daily contact with the patients it had to be they who determined and should determine priorities in the health care sector. There is some misunderstanding here about the values underlying the making of priorities in health care, the possible sources of these values, and the relative legitimacy of different sources. There is further a possible lack of appreciation of the frequent need in any debate about priority setting and the distribution of property rights regarding priority setting to distinguish between technical (informed) judgments and value judgments.

It is of course not to be expected that values in health care will change at the same time, at the same rate or even from the same base in different cultures. Some societies are more likely to have a more technocratic set of values underlying their social structure than others; some will be more receptive to change than others. The same is likely to be true of health care as well and perhaps medicine too.

However a common feature across all developed countries has been the need to cope with at best a slowing in the rate of growth of health services. This has led to greater questioning of the values underlying medicine and with that questioning, some sense of the value of medicine per se, by which we mean what it is that doctors achieve. Most visibly this is seen in the growth of alternative medicine but it is also apparent in the more ready questioning of the dictum that the doctor knows best.

In times of increased relative financial stringency, it is inevitable that questions are asked more vehemently than previously about the relative value of health care vis-à-vis other services competing for society's scarce resources, be they educational facilities, industrial growth or simply private consumption, as citizens become increasingly aware of the effect of a growing tax base on their disposable income. Thus efficiency has become a common expression in health care in the 1980s, even if its acceptance in medicine remains much more limited. Increasingly governments and policy makers more generally have begun to question whether society's resources are being well spent on and within the health care sector. But such questioning cannot go far without at some stage coming up against the medical values which, despite some of the views expressed above, remain somewhat autocratic and remote from the world of limited resources. The limits on resources have in fact pointed more firmly than ever to the limits of medicine. The realisation more clearly that it is *society's* resources that are being consumed by the doctors in the treatment of their patients has inevitably pushed the question of better use of resources beyond health care into the realms of medicine. Doctors cannot act without society's resources and society has increasingly come to recognise this.

There has been a shift in the distribution of property rights in health care which has begun to eat into the medical terrain. Clearly a relevant factor here is the question of improved education in general, but also more specifically, in health and medical matters among the population at large. These factors have facilitated change but we would argue that it is the shift in the economic frame that has been the catalyst.

The medical value base has been further undermined by the doubts that efficiency enquiries have raised about the effectiveness of modern medicine. Studies of efficiency cannot make much headway if they do not address the question of whether and to what extent the various medical treatment practices are doing good. It is just such studies which are revealing not so much that doctors' practices do not do good but rather that since doctors seem to do such very different things or the same things at so many different rates when faced with what appear to be very similar patients, they cannot all be providing the most effective treatment. Of course medicine is an inexact science and of course there is some truth in the notion that no two patients are the same. But there is now no doubt from the evidence accumulated over a wide range of procedures and countries that doctors are doing very different things to comparable patients (McPherson *et al.*, 1982).

Such evidence begins to raise some serious implications for the faith that societies normally place in their medical doctors and in the practice of medicine. We have learned to believe that the most efficient way to protect ourselves against disease is to train a highly specialised cadre of professionals who can provide us with the necessary information and treatments when we are sick to give us the best possible chance to recover. It has become accepted that the patient, ignorant of both his or her health status and what best to do about it, can rely on the highly trained and informed doctor to provide the necessary skills. These basic social assumptions are now open to challenge. The state of medicine is currently perilous.

Given that medicine is an inexact science and that in so far as it is converted even today in many industrialised countries back into something not so far removed from 'witch doctory'—at least as much the wish, the responsibility or even the fault of the population as it is of the doctors—then the evidence of practice variations in itself need not be too worrying. Values do change over time and we can expect that the inexactitudes associated with medicine can become a part of the science of medicine and of the attitudes of society at large as well as individual patients.

What is however of more concern in this area is the slowness and unwillingness of the medical profession to change. This is seen specifically in the context of the slowness of medical education to incorporate the new ideas and values associated with a world that has in many ways come to accept that resources for health care are limited. Too many doctors still qualify without having been exposed to the most elementary teaching in management and economics. Old-fashioned concepts of clinical freedom may be dying in some of the higher and more refined echelons of the profession but they are still alive and well in so many of the fresh young minds coming out of today's medical schools.

But the evidence that doctors are doing so very different things to their similar patients has been around for some time. It is a widespread phenomenon. What is distressing is not the evidence but the lack of response to it from the profession. Yet if the profession does not awake to the need to get it right, or at least for more of them to agree on what is right, then it will be only natural for the cost-containing politicians and administrators to step in and cut resources. And why not, if there is no evidence in certain circumstances that doing more means doing better while it is clearly the case that doing more means greater costs. There is a challenge to the profession there that needs to be picked up but their current defensive and conservative attitude cannot but harm the profession in the longer run and undermine still further the social values on which the strength of the profession is inevitably founded.

But how does the growing awareness that resources are scarce and that health care should be apportioned in a more rational way than has been the case hitherto influence values of health care? How does the changing economic and political climate surrounding health care lead to a change of values in health care?

The recognition that health care cannot be understood and analysed in abstraction from its economic conditions and implications has meant that an ethical approach, utilitarianism (which earlier had only a very limited impact on medicine and the health professions), has come to play a dominant role in recent thinking about medicine and health care. Traditionally, medical doctors and other health professionals have argued or reacted along the lines of deontological ethics, or have been intuitively supporting the moral ideal prescribing responsibility for the weak. The individual patient or client has been the main concern of the professional.

Under the impact of economic reasoning and the calculations of the cost–benefit analyst, a utilitarian approach to value questions paves the way for a new ethical attitude. The professional is now faced with a different value system that suggests that his or her concern for the individual patient may not tally with a concern for the benefit of the greatest number.

Though this utilitarian approach, as advocated by many economists and planners, has come to play a central role in recent discussions about health care, it has not yet come to dominate the practice of health policy. Even more slowly—often not at all—the utilitarian approach has been adopted by professionals. What are the reasons for that?

Firstly, the recognition that economics has to be taken into account in health care has arisen at the same time as patients, patient organisations and many politicians have been strongly reacting against the power and paternalism of professionals, especially medical doctors. There is a demand for stronger consumer influence on health care and its institutions. A grass-roots reaction against bureaucracy and paternalism has stressed the need to let patients' values play a greater role in the distribution and organisation of health care. Grass-roots critics to a large extent agree with generalists (health economists and planners) when pointing to the deficiencies in current health care systems.

On the other hand and at the same time, grass-roots critics of bureaucracy and paternalism have been just as reluctant to accept the ideas of health economists as have many professionals. They have obviously been afraid that the paternalism of the health professionals would be replaced by the paternalism of the generalists who would legitimate cuts in health care budgets and redistribution of health care without allowing the patients to have more influence on the system and its functions.

From the standpoint of liberal democracy this attitude may appear puzzling. The use of cost–benefit analyses should not be interpreted as being in opposition to the relativistic attitude expressed by many critics of today's paternalism. These analyses are simply necessary tools, to be used by politicians before making justified choices among various treatment—and health care—strategies. Having seen the economists' calculations, politicians then make their choices in the light of what they consider to be the dominant values in the population or in accordance with their own personal values which they have laid open to the population. If politicians are to ration health care in ways which do not reflect the values of the electorate, then they can, of course, always be changed at the next election.

This *ideal* picture of politics as an expression of the aggregate values of the individual citizens does not, however, satisfy grass-roots critics of bureaucracy and paternalism in today's welfare systems. Grass-roots critics want patients and citizens in general to have a more direct influence on the welfare system. A more rational basis for political decision making does not in itself provide that.

On the other hand, politicians have not been particularly willing to ration health care. In many countries they seem to favour the traditional practice of leaving doctors to do it. Only rarely are politicians inclined to take the political responsibility for decisions to the effect that a particular kind of treatment in use should be given up or that a new kind of treatment (e.g. transplant surgery) which is technically feasible should not be brought into use.

So, it appears that critics *from below* (grass-roots) and critics *from above* (e.g. health economists) have reached deadlock. This is perhaps part of the explanation why much simpler economic and ideological considerations than the models of health economists have come to play a dominant role in recent controversies about changing welfare systems. Politicians and planners often refer to the critique from the grass-roots opponents (and others) against the paternalistic and bureaucratic dominance of health care.

But a much simpler remedy than the one suggested by health economists is introduced: *the market mechanism*. Even in socialist countries with great problems in organising and distributing health care in an effective and just way, there has been some revival of traditional market thinking. The intention is not primarily (at least not in Scandinavian and socialist countries) to *privatise* health care in general but to make the health care system more efficient in terms of resource use and in accordance with the demands of the consumers, e.g. by letting them 'pay' for the services they prefer, for example, by vouchers.

The recent revival of the market model in many quarters has gone hand in hand with a renaissance of liberal ideology as expressed, for example, in the idea of deontological autonomy. This value change is associated with changing conceptions of disease, as can be seen in the programme for prevention recently published by the Danish Minister of Health. Here it is pointed out that we are now facing a new sickness profile: lifestyle diseases are defined explicitly as being caused by our individual lifestyle or personal habits, so in the long run, citizens should be held responsible for the example of deontological autonomy. To sum up: present attempts to make health care systems more efficient and to find means to ration scarce resources have evoked two antagonistic approaches to value in western culture: the utilitarian and the deontological.

This is, however, only part of the picture of conflicting values in recent discussions about modernisation or restructuring of health care systems in industrialised countries.

Critics of European health care systems have complained not only that the systems are bureaucratic and paternalistic, but also that they have not secured *equity* in health, a criticism which is particularly serious for health care systems of the welfare state variety which are rooted in the optimistic ideology that equal access to health care would lead to equality in health.

In recent years the ideal of equity in health has in many countries been espoused as the basic end of health policy. Equity is also the basic value of the WHO programme *Health for all by the year 2000* (1983) which has been endorsed at least on paper by almost all European countries, and by many governments all over the world.

Equity in health as the basic end of health policy does not mean that all should achieve exactly the same biological, psychological and social condition, whatever that means. What advocates would seem to purport for its meaning is firstly, that at any point in history (within a limited social and cultural context) it is possible to stipulate a health status assumed to be a necessary state for individuals realising their particular ideals and life plans. Secondly, through health policy steps should be taken such that all members of the community can achieve this status.

The problem here, as we see it, is that there is a gap in the logic of the values being applied. Health, as discussed at several points in this volume, is today accepted as a value-laden concept. How it is valued and the extent to which it is valued will vary from individual to individual. Again, the value attached to the consumption of health care will vary from individual to individual. (Two individuals may value some change in health status equally but differ in their assessment of the probability or extent that health care consumption can bring about that change.)

But the extent to which individuals consume health care is a function not just of the values they attach to consumption but the accessibility of that care. Equality of access has consequently become for many health care systems the goal of equity. But equal access, if individuals value consumption of health care differently, will *not* lead to equal utilisation of health care. And if policy were to strive for equal utilisation, in such a case it would require unequal access i.e. what might be called 'positive discrimination'.

What then of equal health? Above we have suggested that there is no reason to believe that equal access will lead to equal utilisation if individuals differ in their valuation of health and/or health care. But would equal utilisation, if it were to be achieved, lead to equal health? Clearly one would want to adjust for need or initial health status here but even then it is unlikely that equal utilisation will lead to equal health. Patients with the same problems respond differently to treatment.

In our view there are thus two 'logical gaps' in the view that equal access will result in equal health. First, equal access will not itself result in equal utilisation; secondly, equal utilisation will not necessarily result in equal health.

What emerges clearly here is the need to assess explicitly what the goals of equity are or should be. To do so needs careful consideration of the ethical and economic implications of the different choices.

Can these different trends in health policy—the deontological approach taken by proponents of the market model, the utilitarianism of economists advocating cost–benefit analyses as a tool for rational health policy—and the widespread more or less intuitive appeal to justice or equity be reconciled?

Is it possible to argue that the shortcomings of health care systems in respect of realising the end of equity of access can be remedied by implementing the market model? We have no empirical reason whatsoever for believing that such a model (e.g. letting the consumers buy health care using vouchers distributed by health authorities) will do so. Quite simply, proponents of the market do not aim at equity.

Will rationing health care on the basis of cost–benefit analyses promote equity? The utilitarian strategies are probably necessary but certainly not sufficient conditions for developing a health policy leading to greater equity. For, as pointed out by Veatch (1981), 'the utilitarian strategy does not take into account the distribution of benefits and harms. It merely examines net aggregate benefits', which implies that if enough people receive the benefits it is plausible that even enormous harms to a small number will be outweighed by the aggregate benefit to the masses'.

Of course Veatch is right if those not suffering 'enormous harms' are not disturbed by the knowledge that health policy is inflicting 'enormous harms to a small number'. So much depends on how we define benefits to the masses. It may be stretching the conventional interpretation of utilitarianism and cost–benefit analysis to take such interdependences into account but certainly with regard to the latter, some economists would want in principle at least to attempt to include the feelings of the masses for the enormously harmed minority to be weighed in the cost–benefit calculus. (One of us, Mooney (1986), has previously argued against Veatch on this point, that it is not just the medical outcome—essentially health—that matters here but for the citizen what it is that he/she wants from his/her health service, for example, the protection of all.)

However a pure or strict utilitarian approach will not *in itself* imply any ethical basis for protecting minorities and weak groups. What is needed is a restructuring of health care systems involving decentralisation and democratisation, making local communities more responsible for the functioning of health care systems while at the same time utilising the resources of weak groups and motivating such groups to take part in the solution of health problems. Perhaps most fundamentally it involves recognising as we have suggested that the utility that citizens gain from their health services (see the discussion of Margolis, 1982, in our opening chapter to this volume) is more than just the 'selfish' utility associated with their own health status but also the utility of knowing that the weak too have the opportunity to have their health status improved.

Distributional issues in health care matter primarily in the context of protecting the weak, but the nature of that protection at a health care level ought not to follow deontological lines. Rather we would argue that social autonomy should dominate health policy; the individual's autonomy ought to be protected at the level of individual choice. What this means in practice is that distribution goals should aim at equality of access and that, with regard to the exercise of patient autonomy, health policy should concentrate on allowing, creating or fostering informed patient choice.

The market ideology fails in health care quite simply because the market fails in health care. That failure is fundamental. Markets cannot work adequately without informed consumers. Patients in many consumption decisions in health care are not informed or at least not sufficiently so. Indeed often what they consume is information.

Classical utilitarianism may also fail if it does not attempt to take account of distributional issues. If cost–benefit analyses ignore these they may fail to reflect the importance (utility or benefit?) that citizens get from knowing that their health service is concerned with distributional issues. That is not a circular argument. Any other simply omits an important source of value in modern health care systems.

REFERENCES

Cochrane, A. L. (1972) *Effectiveness and Efficiency: Random Reflections on Health Services*. Nuffield Provincial Hospitals Trust, London.

Gøtrik, J. K. (1987) *Medical Debat* October: 40.

Hoffenberg, R. (1987) *Clinical Freedom*. Nuffield Provincial Hospitals Trust, London.

Jennett, B. (1983) *High Technology Medicine, Benefits and Burdens*. The Nuffield Provincial Hospitals Trust, London.

Margolis, H. (1982) *Selfishness, Altruism and Rationality*. Cambridge University Press, Cambridge.

McPherson, K., Wennberg, J. E., Hovind, D. B. *et al.* (1982) Small area variations in the use of common surgical procedures: an international comparison. *New England Journal of Medicine* **307**, 1310–14.

Mooney, G. H. (1986) *Economics, Medicine and Health Care*. Wheatsheaf, Brighton.

Veatch, R. M. (1981) *A Theory of Medical Ethics*. Basic Books, New York, pp. 259–60.

WHO (1983) *Targets in Support of the Regional Strategy for Health for All 2000*. WHO/EURO, Copenhagen.

Index

14434996R00117

Made in the USA
San Bernardino, CA
15 December 2018